Withdrawn
from stock
16/4/24

ABC OF MONITORING DRUG THERAPY

ABC OF
MONITORING DRUG THERAPY

J K ARONSON FRCP

Clinical reader in clinical pharmacology, Radcliffe Infirmary, Oxford

M HARDMAN MRCP

Medical adviser, medical research department, Zeneca Pharmaceuticals, Macclesfield

D J M REYNOLDS MRCP

Clinical lecturer in clinical pharmacology, Radcliffe Infirmary, Oxford

Published by the BMJ Publishing Group
Tavistock Square, London WC1H 9JR

First published 1993

British Library Cataloguing in Publication Data

A catalogue record for this book is available
from the British Library

ISBN 0–7279–0791–3

Printed in Great Britain at the University Press, Cambridge
Typesetting by Bedford Typesetters Limited, Bedford

Contents

INTRODUCTION

This book is based on a series of articles which first appeared in the *BMJ*. We wrote the articles in response to requests for information about some of the simple principles underlying the use of plasma or serum concentration measurements of some drugs which are frequently measured in monitoring therapy (for example, when to take a blood sample in relation to the time of drug administration). We also included an article on patient compliance, because of its importance in drug therapy.

Monitoring therapy by measuring plasma drug concentrations has been advocated for many drugs. We have included here the half dozen drugs or groups of drugs for which requests are most commonly made and for which there is the most convincing evidence that their measurement may be of help. We cannot emphasise too much, however, that measurement of drug concentration is only an adjunct to good drug therapy and should be considered in conjunction with other aspects of the patient's condition, never in isolation. In the last chapter we have outlined what we think are the best ways of using the plasma drug concentration measurement to improve drug therapy.

We have included illustrative case histories, taken from clinical practice, to show how drug therapy can go wrong and how measurement of the plasma drug concentration can help to avoid or remedy problems. These histories therefore reflect the problems of clinical practice and should not be regarded as paradigms of good drug therapy.

We are grateful to Deborah Reece of the *BMJ* for her expert help in marshalling the illustrations.

J K Aronson
M Hardman
D J M Reynolds

Oxford and Macclesfield

February 1993

WHY MONITOR DRUG THERAPY?

J K Aronson, M Hardman

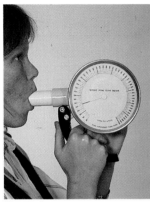

The peak expiratory flow rate in patients with asthma can be used to monitor diurnal variation in airways resistance and the effects of bronchodilators.

It is common clinical practice to monitor the response to treatment of a disease. Obvious examples include monitoring the treatment of hypertension by measuring a patient's blood pressure, the course of an infection by measuring body temperature, and asthma by measuring the peak expiratory flow rate. The effects of a drug are not often monitored, however, despite the fact that monitoring techniques are available. In this book we will discuss:

- The reasons for monitoring drug treatment
- The ways in which therapeutic responses to drugs can be measured
- Monitoring patient compliance
- Measuring and interpreting plasma drug concentrations as a means of monitoring drug treatment.

Why monitor drug treatment?

Reasons for monitoring drug treatment

1 To see whether there is a therapeutic response
2 To assess drug toxicity
3 To assess compliance

The aim of all drug treatment is to improve the patient's condition, and this aim has two parts: to achieve the maximum therapeutic benefit, and to minimise unwanted effects (such as adverse drug reactions and interactions).

Direct or indirect monitoring of drug treatment may allow the doctor to assess the degree of therapeutic response. No response might indicate that the dosage is inadequate, another drug would be better, the diagnosis is incorrect, or the patient has not taken the drug in the manner prescribed.

Monitoring drug treatment is also important to detect adverse effects. In many cases the correct dose of a drug can be found only by initial trial, subsequent monitoring, and consequent adjustment of the dosage regimen. In making adjustments it is important to remember that the dosage regimen includes the dose of the drug, the route and frequency of administration, and the duration of treatment.

Questions in monitoring drug treatment

Examples of easily measurable therapeutic responses

- Urine output in patients treated with desmopressin for diabetes insipidus
- Intraocular pressure in patients treated with timolol eye drops for glaucoma
- Muscle fatigue in patients treated with pyridostigmine for myasthenia gravis

Is there a directly measurable therapeutic response?

Sometimes the direct therapeutic response can be measured easily. In other instances, however, the interpretation of a measurable response is not so clear cut. For example, an apparent response may be due to spontaneous resolution of the disease, as when a viral sore throat improves spontaneously after an antibiotic has been prescribed inappropriately. An absent measureable therapeutic response to a drug, however, usually suggests that either a change in dosage regimen or a different therapeutic approach altogether is required.

Why monitor drug therapy?

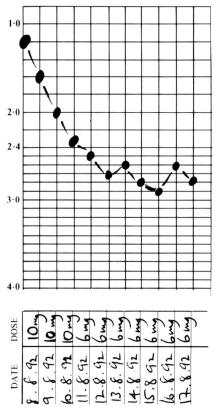

DATE	DOSE
8.6.92	10 mg
9.6.92	10 mg
10.8.92	10 mg
11.6.92	6 mg
12.8.92	6 mg
13.6.92	6 mg
14.8.92	6 mg
15.8.92	6 mg
16.6.92	6 mg
17.8.92	6 mg

Changes in the international normalised ratio (INR) during the initiation of warfarin therapy. Measurement of the INR before the start of treatment and daily during the first few days allows careful planning of appropriate treatment.

Is there a directly measurable response that, although itself not the end point, may be related to the end point?

Measuring the blood pressure in a patient with hypertension indicates whether the blood pressure has fallen satisfactorily with treatment. It will not, however, tell whether that patient is going to have a stroke. Population studies indicate that the risk of having a stroke is reduced by effective treatment, but a doctor never knows in an individual patient whether lowering the blood pressure reduced his or her risk of stroke or of any other complication of hypertension.

In patients who have had a pulmonary embolus and are being treated with warfarin the international normalised ratio (INR) is used to assess the degree of anticoagulation. This allows doctors to use warfarin as safely as possible in terms of preventing, on the one hand, overanticoagulation and an increased risk of bleeding and, on the other hand, underanticoagulation and the further high risk of embolus. For an individual patient, however, the doctor cannot know whether maintaining the international normalised ratio within the accepted therapeutic range will prevent a further pulmonary embolus.

In some cases it may be difficult to differentiate responses to drugs from changes in the disease that are not related to treatment. For example, weight loss in a patient with congestive cardiac failure treated with diuretics may be due to an increase in cardiac output and may therefore indicate a therapeutic response. The weight loss could, however, be due to cachexia. Similarly, a steady weight in such a patient treated long term with diuretics may be due to good control of heart failure but could also result from a combination of weight loss secondary to cachexia and weight gain due to fluid retention.

Examples of effects to monitor if therapeutic outcome cannot be assessed directly

Clinically related effect
—Resolution of fever when pneumococcal pneumonia is treated with benzylpenicillin

Pharmacological effect
—The international normalised ratio (INR) during treatment with warfarin

---

Is the amount of drug in the body appropriate?

Measuring the amount of drug in the body (by measuring the plasma concentration) comes last in the list of priorities for monitoring drug treatment. When possible the therapeutic outcome should be assessed directly. If that is not possible then either a clinically related effect (for example, the resolution of fever when pneumococcal pneumonia is treated with benzylpenicillin) or a pharmacological effect (for example, blood clotting during treatment with anticoagulants) may be measured. This may not always be possible, however, and in some cases measuring the plasma concentration of a drug may provide useful information about the adequacy of the dosage regimen or the likelihood of toxicity.

Conclusion

Monitoring the effects of drugs is an essential part of therapy. Where possible look for the therapeutic or toxic effects of the drug; otherwise try to measure its pharmacological action or plasma concentration

---

It can never be assumed that treating a patient with a given drug will produce the desired effect. The onus is on the prescribing doctor to follow the patient's progress and to monitor the response to that drug. Only by monitoring the effect of the drug by the most appropriate means available can the optimum therapeutic response be achieved.

PATIENT COMPLIANCE

J K Aronson, M Hardman

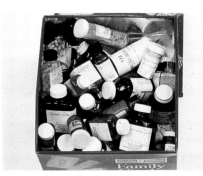

Patients don't always take their drugs in the recommended fashion. This tin contains drugs belonging to a patient and his wife; there are several full bottles of warfarin, antibiotics, and a range of psychotropic drugs.

Doctors assume that when they give a patient a prescription the drug will be taken as directed. But patients do not always take their prescribed drugs, and if there is no therapeutic response to a given dosage regimen poor compliance must be considered. Hippocrates warned that patients may often lie about taking their medicines.

Up to 20% of patients fail to collect their prescribed drugs within one month of issue and are therefore non-compliant from the start.[1] Even patients who collect their drugs may not take them. Rates of compliance have been variously estimated at between 10% and 90% and depend on many factors, including the enthusiasm of the doctor, the disease being treated, and the patient's perception of the importance of the disease.[2]

Methods of assessing compliance

Method	Description	Comments
Methods of assessing compliance		
Tablet counting		
Discrepancy count	The number of tablets dispensed is known, the remaining tablets are counted	Patient is aware of observation and may dispose of remaining tablets
Discrepancy estimate	The number of tablets dispensed is known, the patient is asked whether any more are required before the next visit	Patient is not aware of being closely observed but the count is less accurate
Recording devices		
Medication monitor	A uranium source and photographic film record the regularity with which the drug is removed	Primarily used in research. Both methods presuppose that the removal of the drug implies that the drug has been taken
Silicon chip recorder	A silicon chip recorder is incorporated into the bottle cap and activated whenever the cap is removed	
Measuring drug or added compound in plasma/urine/faeces		
Drug	The concentration of drug is measured directly— for example, plasma phenytoin concentration	Variations may be due to pharmacokinetic differences and not compliance. Primarily used in research. May be misleading if the drug is taken only on the day of measurement
Inert marker	A compound such as phenobarbitone, riboflavin, or phenol red is incorporated into the drug formulation and can be measured in the urine	
Colour changes	For example, iron colours faeces black, rifampicin turns urine red	
Measuring pharmacological effect		
	For example, pupil size with pilocarpine, exercise heart rate with β adrenoceptor antagonists	

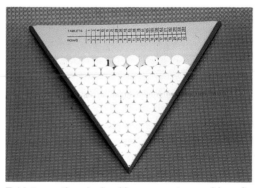

Tablet counting device. You may get some idea of compliance by counting the number of tablets in the bottle and comparing this with the prescribed number of tablets.

Caron and Roth showed that doctors could not predict their patients' compliance more accurately than by chance[3]; so if compliance is to be accurately assessed specific methods must be used. Direct questioning can sometimes be useful in establishing whether a patient is compliant. Patients are more willing to admit defaulting if questioned tactfully—for example, "Have you managed to take all the tablets?" rather than "Have you missed any tablets?" Having an objective means of assessing compliance may be very helpful in difficult cases and is vital in drug trials. Methods of assessing compliance include:

- Tablet counting
- Recording devices
- Measuring the concentration of the drug in body fluids
- Measuring a marker substance added to the drug
- Measuring the pharmacological effect.

3

Methods of improving compliance

Each 0.5 ml contains:
Fluphenazine Decanoate B.P.   12.5 mg
in Sesame Oil Ph. Eur.
Preservative:
Benzyl Alcohol Ph. Eur.   1.5%
Sterile
For deep intramuscular injection only

Some medicines are formulated in special oils. After deep intramuscular injection the drug is released slowly into the body over a few weeks. Compliance with medication can thus be ensured by regular administration in the outpatient department.

Compliance may be improved in four ways.

(1) *By ensuring compliance*

- A single dose can be given by the doctor or nurse—for example, gonorrhoea can be treated by a single intramuscular dose of procaine penicillin

- A depot formulation suitable for implantation or intramuscular injection can be given at specified regular intervals in the outpatient department—for example, in the treatment of schizophrenia fluphenazine decanoate is given as a depot intramuscular injection at regular intervals (for example, fortnightly)

- The patient can be supervised while taking the drug—for example, during treatment in hospital, by parents giving medicines to their children, visitors giving drugs to relatives, and a district nurse giving medicines to elderly people.

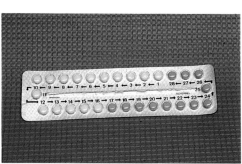

Calendar packs remind patients when to take their medicines.

(2) *By removing barriers to compliance*

- The palatability of medicines can be improved—for example, by flavouring medicines for children (such as banana flavoured antibiotics) or by using slow release formulations to prevent unpalatable medicines from being tasted (such as potassium chloride)

- Elixirs can be used instead of tablets, especially in young children or in elderly people, who might have difficulty in swallowing large tablets. Examples of drugs which may successfully be given in this way are potassium chloride, digoxin, and benorylate

- If a certain formulation causes adverse effects change to another—for example, if ferrous sulphate causes diarrhoea slow release iron formulations can be tried, although iron given in this way may be less effective

- Blister calendar packs for oral contraceptives or β blockers help patients to remember to take the drug.

Examples of useful combinations of drugs
- Iron with folic acid during pregnancy
- Rifampicin with isoniazid in tuberculosis
- A thiazide with a potassium sparing diuretic in heart failure

---

(3) *By simplifying therapeutic regimens*

(a) By reducing the number of tablets a patient has to take

(b) By reducing the frequency of administration.

It may be possible to reduce the number of tablets a patient has to take by avoiding or discontinuing unnecessary drugs and by using a combination of drugs in a single tablet. The chief disadvantage of combined formulations is that the individual drug dosages cannot be adjusted.

A reduction in the frequency of administration can be achieved by using so called modified release formulations. Examples include modified release theophylline formulations for asthma and modified release morphine for chronic pain. Another means of reducing the frequency of administration is to use a larger dose than usual given less frequently. High dose ampicillin for urinary tract infections is a good example. Two doses of 3 g are as effective as a seven day course.

Tailoring drug dosages to the individual patient to minimise adverse effects is especially important in prophylaxis and in asymptomatic conditions such as hypertension and hyperlipidaemia.

Examples of bad combinations of drugs
- Potassium with diuretics
- Amitriptyline 12·5 mg with chlordiazepoxide 5 mg

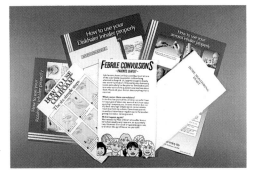

There are many information leaflets available to help patients take their drugs.

Patients bringing tablets at each visit presents opportunities for:

- Making sure that patients have all the drugs they should have and in the correct strengths
- Demonstrating the correct method of using an inhaler
- Ensuring that glyceryl trinitrate is kept in a dark bottle with a foil lined cap and no cotton wool padding
- Monitoring compliance

(4) *By educating the patient*

Educating patients about the nature of their condition and the necessity and aims of treatment is known to improve compliance in certain conditions (for example, glaucoma and diabetes mellitus). Patients' perception of their own health, however, may be more important than how well they understand their underlying illness, and there is evidence that intensive education programmes do not necessarily improve compliance.[4] None the less, education of the patient is always to be encouraged, and if it does improve compliance then so much the better.

Compliance can also be improved to some extent by rewarding compliant patients with praise and by reminding and encouraging patients whose compliance is poor. Patients can also be helped by information leaflets, such as have been proposed by the Royal Pharmaceutical Society for eye drops, eye ointments, ear drops, nose drops, pessaries, and suppositories.

All patients should be encouraged to bring their tablets with them at each visit as this allows the doctor to know exactly what drugs the patient is taking, to identify precisely any drugs that the patient could not otherwise tell him or her about or whose dosage is uncertain, and (to some extent) to monitor compliance. Having the tablets in front of you can be very helpful in sorting out some of the practical aspects of drug treatment.

Other ways of helping

Finally, patients usually find it helpful to have a clearly written list of their current drugs with dosages and frequency of administration. Clear labelling on medicine bottles also helps.

1 Rashid A. Do patients cash prescriptions? *BMJ* 1982;**284**:24-6.
2 Griffith S. A review of the factors associated with patient compliance and the taking of prescribed medicines. *Br J Gen Prac* 1990;**40**:114-6.
3 Caron HS, Roth HP. Patients' cooperation with a medical regimen. Difficulties in identifying the noncooperator. *JAMA* 1968;**203**:922-6.
4 Sackett DL, Haynes RB, Gibson ES, Hackett BC, Taylor DW, Roberts RS, *et al.* Randomised clinical trial of strategies for improving medication compliance in primary hypertension. *Lancet* 1975;i:1205-7.

MEASURING PLASMA DRUG CONCENTRATIONS

J K Aronson, M Hardman

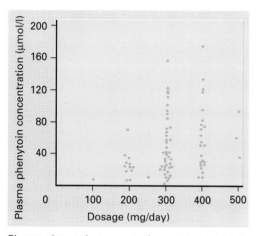

Plasma phenytoin concentrations at steady state in relation to total daily dose. At all dosages there are large variations in mean steady state concentration from subject to subject.

Factors that modify drug plasma concentration for a given dose

- Drug formulation
- Drug interactions
- Environmental factors
- Genetic variation
- Renal and hepatic function

If a given dose of a drug produced the same plasma concentration in all patients there would be no need to measure the plasma concentration of the drug. However, people vary considerably in the extent to which they absorb, distribute, and eliminate drugs. Tenfold or even greater differences in steady state plasma concentrations have been found among patients treated with the same dose of important drugs such as phenytoin, warfarin, and digoxin. The following are some of the many reasons for these differences.

Formulation—Some drugs—for example, digoxin—are better absorbed from liquid formulations than from tablets. Phenytoin toxicity has been reported after a chemical change in a supposedly inert excipient (calcium sulphate to lactose) in phenytoin capsules.

Genetic variation—For example, in some people drugs are acetylated slowly, in others they are acetylated quickly. Drugs whose metabolism is affected by acetylation include hydralazine, procainamide, and isoniazid.

Environmental variation—For example, smoking increases the rate of clearance of theophylline.

Effects of disease—The pharmacokinetics of some drugs may be altered by disease—for example, renal impairment decreases the rate of elimination of gentamicin, digoxin, and lithium. In patients with hepatic disease the metabolism of drugs such as phenytoin and carbamazepine may be reduced, resulting in increased plasma concentrations.

Drug interactions—For example, quinidine and verapamil increase the plasma concentration of digoxin by interfering with its renal elimination; diuretics increase the plasma concentration of lithium by interfering with its renal excretion.

Measuring the plasma concentration of a drug allows the doctor to tailor the dosage to the individual patient and to obtain the maximum therapeutic effect with minimal risk of toxicity.

Clinical usefulness

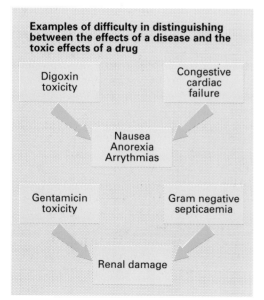

Examples of difficulty in distinguishing between the effects of a disease and the toxic effects of a drug

Digoxin toxicity / Congestive cardiac failure → Nausea Anorexia Arrythmias

Gentamicin toxicity / Gram negative septicaemia → Renal damage

There is only a small number of drugs for which measuring the plasma concentration is helpful in clinical practice. The following criteria must be satisfied for the plasma concentration of a drug to be useful.

(1) *Difficulty in interpreting clinical evidence of therapeutic or toxic effects*—If it is easy to measure the therapeutic or toxic effects of a drug directly the plasma drug concentration gives little additional information about drug action—for example, there is little point in measuring the plasma insulin concentration in a diabetic patient as blood glucose measurements give a direct indication of the short term action of the drug. On the other hand, it is difficult to measure the therapeutic effects of phenytoin, and measuring the plasma concentration helps to tailor the dose within the appropriate therapeutic range.

Occasionally it may be difficult to distinguish between the effects of a disease and the toxic effects of a drug—for example, renal failure may occur in a patient with a Gram negative septicaemia, either because of the disease or because of an adverse effect of the gentamicin used to treat it; both congestive cardiac failure and digoxin toxicity may produce nausea, anorexia, and arrhythmias. In these cases the plasma drug concentration will provide important information that is not obtainable by any other means and will allow appropriate alterations in drug dosages to be made.

Measuring plasma drug concentrations

Measurement of proved value
Aminoglycoside antibiotics
Anticonvulsants:
    Phenytoin
    Carbamazepine
Digoxin and digitoxin
Lithium
Theophylline
Cyclosporin
Thyroid hormones
Cycloserine
Flucytosine
Vancomycin

Sometimes measured but case not proved
Antiarrhythmic drugs:
    Lignocaine
    Procainamide
    Quinidine
    Amiodarone
Anticonvulsants other than phenytoin and carbamazepine
Methotrexate
Tricyclic antidepressants
Itraconazole

(2) *A good relation between the plasma concentration of a drug and either its therapeutic or its toxic effect*—There is little point in measuring the plasma drug concentration if it will not give interpretable information about the therapeutic or toxic state of the patient—for example, if there is a subtherapeutic concentration of digoxin in a patient with compensated heart failure with sinus rhythm digoxin may be withdrawn without fear that the patient's heart failure will worsen; a high peak concentration of gentamicin is associated with toxic effects and prompts early adjustments to dosage.

(3) *A low toxic to therapeutic ratio*—Though there are several drugs for which the first two criteria apply, measurement of the plasma concentration may not be useful for them all—for example, while in some cases there may be a good relation between the plasma concentration of penicillin and its therapeutic effect, the dosage range over which penicillin is safe is so large that very high dosages can be given safely. On the other hand, for some drugs (such as lithium, gentamicin, phenytoin, and digoxin) there is only a small difference between the concentrations that are associated with therapeutic effects and those associated with toxic effects.

(4) *The drug should not be metabolised to active metabolites.*—Even if a drug satisfies the three criteria above interpretation of the plasma drug concentration may be rendered difficult by the presence of metabolites with therapeutic or toxic activity. If active metabolites are produced both the parent drug and the metabolites would have to be measured to provide a comprehensive picture of the relation between the total plasma concentration of active compounds and the clinical effect. This is usually not possible in routine monitoring and limits the usefulness of plasma concentration measurements of, for example, procainamide, which is metabolised to N-acetylprocainamide (acecainide), which has equipotent antiarrhythmic activity.

Therapeutic range

Factors that modify the effect of the drug for a given drug plasma concentration

- Drug interactions
- Electrolyte balance
- Acid-base balance
- Age
- Bacterial resistance
- Protein binding (if total concentration measured)

Laboratories quote reference ranges for biochemical measurements. The reference range is the range of values which encompasses 95% of the values found in a large number of healthy people.

There is an analogous method of expression for plasma drug concentration—the therapeutic range. This is derived from measurements in large numbers of patients in carefully controlled studies and is the range within which a therapeutic effect is expected to occur with a minimal risk of toxicity. For example, longitudinal studies in patients with generalised seizures have shown improved seizure control when the plasma phenytoin concentration is increased above 40 µmol/l, and as clinical signs of toxicity increase in frequency at concentrations above 80 µmol/l, 40-80 µmol/l is the therapeutic range.

By analogy with the concept of a reference range the therapeutic range is often assumed to apply to all patients in all circumstances. However, this may not always be so. For example, plasma phenytoin concentrations below 40 µmol/l are sufficient to achieve complete control of seizures in some patients with relatively mild epilepsy while some patients may require concentrations above 80 µmol/l.

A further consideration is that there are often features which are specific to an individual patient and which may alter his or her therapeutic range. The therapeutic range is derived from studies of populations and provides only a guide to those concentrations that may be expected to be associated with a therapeutic effect and to the concentrations above which toxic effects may occur. The tailoring of drug dosages to an individual must take into account those features that are unique to that person, including relevant biochemical measurements and clinical factors.

Obviously a patient who is taking phenytoin and who exhibits classic signs of toxicity, such as nystagmus and ataxia, requires a reduction in the dose regardless of whether the plasma concentration is within the therapeutic range.

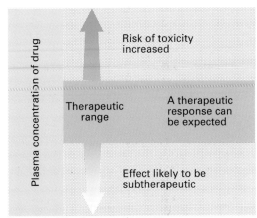

Concept of the therapeutic range.

Measuring plasma drug concentrations

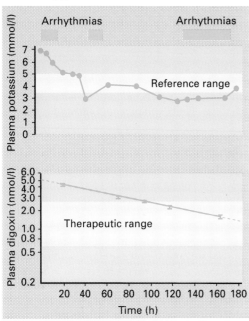

Plasma potassium and digoxin concentrations in a patient after a single intravenous dose of digoxin 0·5 mg. Arrhythmias occurred when the digoxin concentration was high or the potassium concentration low.

Factors that modify the therapeutic range

If the effect of a drug at its site of action is altered for a given concentration the therapeutic range will change. Factors that may alter this concentration-response relation include:

Electrolyte balance—For example, the effects of many antiarrhythmic drugs (such as lignocaine, quinidine, and procainamide) are altered in the presence of hypokalaemia, as are the effects of digoxin.

Acid-base balance—For example, acidosis enhances the effect of digoxin.

Age—For example, there is increased sensitivity to digitalis in elderly people.

Bacterial resistance—For example, although the plasma concentration of gentamicin may be adequate, an organism that is resistant to gentamicin will not be affected.

Plasma protein binding—It is usual when measuring plasma drug concentrations to measure the total amount of drug in the plasma (that is, protein bound and unbound drug). However, the therapeutic effect is largely determined by the unbound concentration. If protein binding changes, the ratio of bound to unbound drug will change, and this will alter the interpretation of the plasma concentration of total drug (this is discussed more fully in the article on phenytoin).

Timing of measurements

Calculation of the length of time it takes to reach steady state

Example

Digoxin has a half life of about 40 hours in a patient with normal renal function. If treatment is given by a daily maintenance dose without an initial loading dose it will take 5×40 hours, or about eight days to achieve steady state

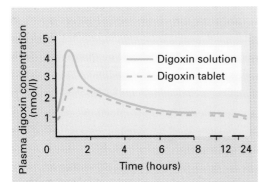

Plasma digoxin concentrations during the 24 h after a single dose during daily maintenance dose therapy. In the 6 h after administration the concentration is a poor guide to the mean steady state concentration.

How long after starting treatment should the plasma concentration be measured?

If you give a drug repeatedly it will accumulate in the body. Eventually, when the amount being given is equal to the amount being eliminated an equilibrium or "steady state" is reached. The time required to reach this steady state depends only on the half life of the drug. After five half lives over 95% of a drug will have accumulated, and for practical purposes steady state can be considered to have been achieved.

The plasma concentration can be measured before this steady state has been reached, but the timing of the sample will have to be taken into consideration when interpreting the result.

How long after the last dose should the sample be taken?

It is preferable to have a sample that reflects the mean steady state concentration during a dosage interval. If the sample is taken too soon after the last dose (for example, at the time of the peak or maximum steady state concentration) it will not have the mean concentration. It is usually simplest to take a sample just before the next dose is due, as this is a reliable measure of the minimum steady state concentration (a "trough" concentration), even though it slightly underestimates the mean steady state concentration. For aminoglycoside antibiotics both peak and trough concentrations are important.

In subsequent chapters we will discuss individual drugs and show how these basic principles apply to each.

The sources of the data shown in the graphs are W D Hooper *et al, Aust N Z J Med* 1974;4:449 for plasma phenytoin concentrations *v* dosage; J K Aronson, D G Grahame-Smith, *Br J Clin Pharmacol* 1976;3:1045-57 for plasma potassium and digoxin concentrations *v* time; and Lloyd *et al, Am J Cardiol* 1978;42:129-36 for plasma digoxin concentration *v* time. The data are reproduced with the permission of the journals.

DIGOXIN

J K Aronson, M Hardman

Digoxin is a cardiac glycoside extracted from foxgloves. It is used in the treatment of atrial fibrillation with a fast ventricular rate. It is also used in congestive cardiac failure with sinus rhythm, although for this its use is controversial

The plasma digoxin concentration that will result from a given dose of the drug can be predicted at best with only 34% accuracy, although knowledge of a previous concentration improves the ability to predict subsequent concentrations. In outpatients taking a fixed daily dosage, steady state plasma digoxin concentrations vary widely (between 0·5 and 3·5 nmol/l). This means that if a target plasma digoxin concentration is desirable, measuring the concentration may be useful in tailoring dosages to individual requirements.

In this chapter we apply to digoxin the criteria (described in the previous chapter on measuring plasma drug concentrations) which must be fulfilled in part or in full before the measurement of its plasma concentration can be considered worth while.

Criteria for measurement

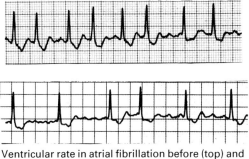

Ventricular rate in atrial fibrillation before (top) and after (bottom) taking digoxin.

Is there difficulty in interpreting clinical evidence of the therapeutic or toxic effects?

In patients with atrial fibrillation the slowing of the ventricular rate is usually a good guide to the therapeutic effect of digoxin. However, in patients with congestive cardiac failure with sinus rhythm who are taking digoxin for its positive inotropic effect there is no easily measurable end point by which to assess the therapeutic response. Furthermore, digoxin toxicity can be difficult to diagnose because anorexia, nausea and vomiting, mental confusion, and cardiac arrhythmias may all be signs or symptoms of both congestive cardiac failure and digitalis toxicity. Thus measuring the plasma digoxin concentration will allow the dosage to be increased within safe limits in order to ensure, firstly, that an adequate response to treatment is not missed because the dose is suboptimal and, secondly, that toxicity does not occur because of too large a dose. Of course this assumes that there is a good relation between the plasma concentration of digoxin and its therapeutic or toxic effects.

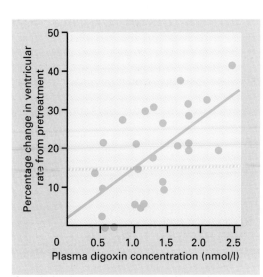

Correlation between percentage change in ventricular rate in atrial fibrillation and plasma digoxin concentration.

Is there a good relation between the plasma concentration and its therapeutic or toxic effects?

In the case of atrial fibrillation there is good evidence that increasing the concentration of digoxin within the therapeutic range produces an increase in its effect of slowing the ventricular rate.

In patients with heart failure in sinus rhythm a relation between the plasma concentration of digoxin and its therapeutic effect has not been clearly established. Generally a satisfactory therapeutic response is most likely to be achieved when plasma digoxin concentrations are between 1·0 nmol/l and 3·8 nmol/l. These limits are based, at least in part, on observations outside this range: the risk of digoxin toxicity increases at concentrations above 2·6 nmol/l and is almost invariable at concentrations greater than 3·8 nmol/l, and it is difficult to detect any effect of digoxin when the plasma concentration is below 1·0 nmol/l. Within the range 1·0 to 3·8 nmol/l there is some evidence of dose responsiveness.

Although concentration correlates well with some measurable actions of digoxin on the heart, such as changes in systolic time intervals and changes in the electrocardiographic configuration (shortened PR interval, prolonged QT_c interval, T wave depression and inversion), these changes are difficult to interpret in terms of the therapeutic outcome.

Digoxin

Therapeutic range
- Below 1 nmol/l a therapeutic effect is unlikely
- Above 3·8 nmol/l the risk of toxicity increases considerably
- Between 1 and 3·8 nmol/l a beneficial effect with a low risk of toxicity is likely

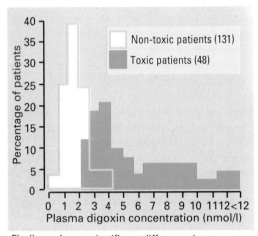

Findings show a significant difference between plasma digoxin concentrations in toxic and non-toxic patients. However, as there is an overlap in the region between about 2 and 3·8 nmol/l the diagnosis cannot be based on a patient's plasma concentration alone.

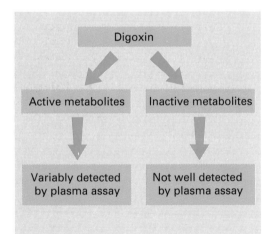

Most studies have shown a significant difference between the mean plasma digoxin concentration in groups of patients with toxicity and the mean concentration in groups without toxicity. The chief problem lies in making the diagnosis of digoxin toxicity in the individual patient. There is no doubt that the plasma concentration on its own is not always sufficient in deciding whether or not a patient has digoxin toxicity. The decision can be made only by considering the plasma digoxin concentration in the light of other clinical and biochemical information. Toxicity is likely when:

- The plasma digoxin concentration is greater than 3·8 nmol/l
- The plasma digoxin concentration is less than 3·8 nmol/l and the plasma potassium concentration is less than 3·5 mmol/l
- The plasma digoxin concentration is less than 3·8 nmol/l and there are any two of the following:
  Plasma potassium >5 mmol/l
  Plasma creatinine >150 μmol/l
  Age >60 years
  Daily maintenance dose >6 μg/kg (for example, 375 μg for a 60 kg patient)

Thus in a patient suspected of having toxicity the plasma potassium and digoxin concentrations and any factors which may alter the patient's sensitivity to digoxin should be considered. If these all support the diagnosis of toxicity the digoxin should be stopped. If the diagnosis is still in doubt the patient should be carefully observed while continuing to take digoxin, but the situation must be reviewed and digoxin should be stopped if necessary. It is certainly better to withhold digoxin from a patient who does not have toxicity than to continue treatment in a patient who does.

For children over 1 year of age the same plasma concentrations are associated with toxicity as in adults. In infants and neonates, however, there is no clear cut pattern and plasma digoxin concentrations can be difficult to interpret.

Is digoxin metabolised to active metabolites?

Most patients metabolise less than 20% of digoxin, and so active metabolites are relatively unimportant. However, about 10% of patients metabolise up to 55%, both by hydrolysis to digoxigenin and to its bisdigitoxosides and monodigitoxosides, all of which have pharmacological activity, and by reduction to dihydrodigoxin, which is relatively inactive. This conversion is thought to occur in the bowel through an effect of gut bacteria, and in those patients in whom it occurs digoxin metabolism may be reduced by antibiotics such as erythromycin and tetracyclines.

In theory, if digoxin metabolism was assayed by measuring the pharmacological activity of all the components (both digoxin and its metabolites) the variation in digoxin would not be a problem. But the types of immunoassay routinely used do not necessarily measure all the metabolites, and in certain cases might give a spuriously low plasma concentration of active cardiac glycosides. This may explain some cases of digoxin toxicity in patients with plasma concentrations in the therapeutic range.

Measurement techniques

All routine laboratories use immunoassay to measure plasma digoxin concentrations, and most use radioimmunoassay with digoxin antibody and an iodine-125 digoxin conjugate as a tracer. This is available in a kit and is relatively easy to use. The problem, as with all immunoassays, is that the antibody may cross react with other compounds. In this case examples include steroid hormones such as cortisol and drugs such as spironolactone. There is also evidence that the serum from neonates, pregnant women, and patients with chronic renal failure and essential hypertension may cross react with digoxin antibody—so called endogenous digitalis-like immunoreactivity. Some antibodies are more susceptible to cross reaction than others.

Antibodies used in digoxin immunoassays are susceptible to cross reaction with other substances.

Factors affecting concentration

Factors which can alter the plasma digoxin concentration when the dosage is kept constant include altered absorption, altered excretion by the kidney, and drug interactions. For example, if renal function is impaired digoxin will be retained and the plasma digoxin concentration will increase without a change in dosage. Similarly, if another drug reduces the rate of elimination of digoxin (such as verapamil, quinidine, or amiodarone) the plasma digoxin concentration will increase.

> **Factors which can increase the plasma digoxin concentration for a given dosage of digoxin include:**
> - Increased absorption due to change of formulation
> - Impaired excretion—for example, impairment of renal function
> - Drug interactions—for example, verapamil, quinidine, and amiodarone
> - Impaired metabolism by antibiotics in people in whom significant metabolism of digoxin occurs in the gut

Factors affecting interpretation

Knowing the plasma digoxin concentration alone is not sufficient for optimal treatment. Several factors change the tissue response to digoxin and must be taken into consideration when interpreting plasma concentrations.

> **Factors which *increase* tissue sensitivity to digoxin include:**
> - Hypokalaemia (for example, due to diuretics)
> - Hypercalcaemia
> - Hypothyroidism
> - Hypoxia and acidosis
>
> **Factors which *decrease* tissue sensitivity to digoxin include:**
> - Hyperkalaemia
> - Hypocalcaemia
> - Hyperthyroidism
> - Neonates

Electrolyte disturbances—Hypokalaemia is the most important and commonest factor which increases the sensitivity of the tissues to digoxin. A reduction in plasma potassium concentration from 3·5 to 3·0 mmol/l is accompanied by an increase in sensitivity to digoxin of about 50%. This is such an important factor that the plasma potassium concentration should always be measured with the plasma digoxin concentration. If the potassium concentration is low digoxin toxicity should be assumed without waiting for the plasma digoxin measurement. Hypercalcaemia and hypomagnesaemia may also be associated with increased tissue sensitivity to digoxin, but the available data are more difficult to interpret.

Thyroid disease—Hypothyroidism increases tissue sensitivity and hyperthyroidism decreases it. This makes interpretation of the plasma digoxin concentration very difficult in patients with thyroid disease.

Age—Elderly people may be more sensitive to digoxin's effects, possibly because of reduced activity of Na^+/K^+ ATPase. However, current dosages and therapeutic guidelines for plasma concentrations are mostly based on studies in elderly people.

Use of plasma measurements

> **Case history: problems associated with renal failure**
>
> A 55 year old man with chronic renal failure (creatinine clearance 50 ml/min) and hypertension was admitted with heart failure. He was found to have atrial fibrillation with a ventricular rate of 170 beats/min. After a loading dose of 500 µg of digoxin his ventricular rate fell to 120 beats/min. With a maintenance dose of 125 µg daily it was still 120 beats/min. His steady state plasma digoxin concentration was 1·6 nmol/l. His daily digoxin dosage was increased by 62·5 µg (50%), which slowed the ventricular rate to 95 beats/min and his plasma digoxin concentration rose predictably to 2·4 nmol/l.
>
> *Conclusion*
>
> Giving the appropriate dosage of digoxin for the degree of renal impairment did not control the patient's ventricular rate. Knowing the plasma digoxin concentration allowed the digoxin dosage to be increased with minimum risk of toxicity.

If the steady state plasma digoxin concentration is known the change in dosage required to change the plasma digoxin concentration by a given amount can be calculated. A given percentage increase in the digoxin dosage will result in the same percentage increase in the steady state plasma concentration. For example, if a patient is taking 250 µg digoxin daily and has a steady state plasma digoxin concentration of 1·2 nmol/l, a daily dosage of 375 (250+125) µg will result in a plasma concentration of 1·8 (1·2+0·6) mmol/l. Thus we can calculate whether a given dosage increase will result in a plasma concentration within or above the therapeutic range.

In practice it is best to aim for a plasma digoxin concentration of 1·0-2·0 nmol/l in the first instance, raising the target carefully to a maximum of 3·0 nmol/l if a therapeutic response is not achieved.

Digoxin

Case history: increased sensitivity to digoxin

A 69 year old woman was admitted with general malaise, anorexia, vomiting, and confusion. She had a history of congestive cardiac failure and had been taking a thiazide diuretic and digoxin 250 µg daily. Her general practitioner had measured her plasma digoxin concentration two days before at 1·6 nmol/l. On admission her serum potassium concentration was 2·9 mmol/l. Correction of the hypokalaemia produced a considerable improvement in all of her original symptoms. She was discharged taking the same dose of digoxin and a combination formulation containing a thiazide diuretic and a potassium sparing diuretic.

Conclusion

This case illustrates two problems: firstly, the difficulty in interpreting a plasma digoxin concentration without the serum potassium concentration, and, secondly, the patient's increased sensitivity to digoxin in the presence of hypokalaemia, which resulted in digoxin toxicity despite a plasma digoxin concentration within the therapeutic range.

Case history: decreased tissue sensitivity to digoxin

A 70 year old man was admitted with congestive cardiac failure and rapid atrial fibrillation. His serum urea and electrolyte concentrations were normal. He was treated with intravenous frusemide 80 mg and oral digoxin 1·25 mg in three divided doses six hours apart. Although his cardiac failure improved slightly, his ventricular rate was still 150 beats/min. His plasma digoxin concentration was 2·2 nmol/l. No further digoxin was given and he was treated with amiodarone. His ventricular rate fell to 90 beats/min and his cardiac failure resolved. His serum triiodothyronine concentration was considerably raised at 8·0 µmol/l. He was treated with carbimazole and when euthyroid underwent successful cardioversion. The amiodarone and diuretics were stopped.

Conclusion

Hyperthyroidism decreases tissue sensitivity to digoxin. The atrial fibrillation did not respond to digoxin in the presence of an apparently adequate plasma digoxin concentration. A further increase in the dosage would probably have resulted in digoxin toxicity without a therapeutic response, but this was avoided by knowing the plasma digoxin concentration. It was also important to withdraw digoxin when amiodarone was introduced as amiodarone increases the plasma digoxin concentration.

Timing of measurements

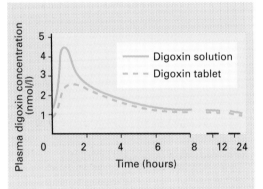

Take the blood sample at least six hours after the last dose of digoxin—the plasma concentration will not necessarily be representative of the true steady state concentration if it is taken earlier.

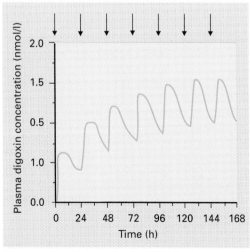

Because digoxin has a long half life it takes several days of regular maintenance dose therapy before a steady state is reached. Arrows indicate when the drug was given.

If you suspect digoxin toxicity or if there is hypokalaemia, withhold digoxin without waiting for the result of the plasma concentration.

There are two aspects to be considered in the timing of blood sampling for plasma digoxin concentrations.

(1) The time after a dose

The plasma digoxin concentration peaks at about one hour after the dose and is at a minimum (trough concentration) just before the next dose. At steady state the logarithmic mean of these measurements is the average steady state concentration, which occurs at about 11 hours after the dose. In practice, the blood sample should be taken at least six hours and preferably 12 hours after the previous dose. This can cause problems in the clinic or practice if the dose of digoxin has been taken in the morning, and patients should therefore be advised to take their digoxin in the evening, as the blood sample may then be taken at any time the next day.

(2) The time it takes during repeated dosage to reach steady state

Measuring the plasma digoxin concentration before a steady state concentration is reached will underestimate the steady state concentration. For example, if a patient takes a daily maintenance dose of digoxin without an initial loading dose it will take about five half lives of digoxin before a steady state is reached. Thus, assuming the patient has normal renal function, it will take 5×40 hours (eight days) to reach a steady state. Of course it may be necessary to measure the plasma digoxin concentration before a steady state is reached if there are concerns about the possibility of digoxin toxicity.

The sources of the data presented in the graphs are: Redfors, *Br Heart J* 1972;**34**:383-91 for change in ventricular rate *v* plasma digoxin concentration; Smith, Haber, *J Clin Invest* 1970;**49**:2377-86 for plasma digoxin concentrations in toxic and non-toxic patients; Lloyd *et al*, *Am J Cardiol* 1978;**42**:129-36 for plasma digoxin concentration *v* time; and J K Aronson, PHD thesis for digoxin reaching steady state. The data are reproduced with permission of the journals.

PHENYTOIN

J K Aronson, M Hardman, D J M Reynolds

Phenytoin is an anticonvulsant whose main use is as a second line drug in treating generalised tonic-clonic seizures and sometimes other forms of epilepsy. It can be used either to treat patients in whom seizures have occurred or to prevent seizures in patients at risk (for example, after neurosurgery).

Because of large individual variation in the disposition of phenytoin patients taking the same dosage have up to a 50-fold difference in plasma phenytoin concentration.

The metabolism of phenytoin is non-linear within the therapeutic range. This is because the enzyme system responsible gradually becomes saturated at relatively low plasma phenytoin concentrations (within the therapeutic range), resulting in a progressive decrease in the rate of elimination of phenytoin as the dosage is increased. As saturation of the enzyme system is reached a small increase in dosage will result in a large increase in plasma phenytoin concentration. Thus, measuring the plasma phenytoin concentration will allow the dosage to be increased within safe limits—ensuring, firstly, that an inadequate response to treatment is not missed because the dose is suboptimal and, secondly, that toxicity does not occur because the dose is too large, which is especially important as the saturation of phenytoin metabolism is approached.

In this chapter we apply to phenytoin the criteria that must be fulfilled in part or in full before the measurement of its plasma concentration can be considered worth while.

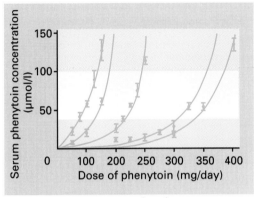

Serum phenytoin concentrations increase non-linearly with increases in dosage.

Criteria for measurement

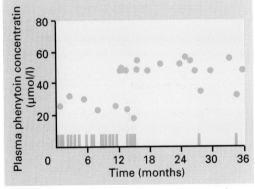

The good relation between plasma concentration and the therapeutic effect of phenytoin is shown by the reduction in seizures (vertical lines) at higher concentrations in this woman.

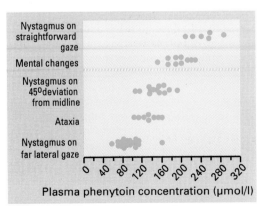

There is a good relation between plasma concentration and the adverse effects of phenytoin.

Is there difficulty in interpreting clinical evidence of the therapeutic or toxic effects?

In patients who are having frequent regular epileptic seizures the total suppression or a measurable reduction in the frequency of seizures is a clearly defined end point by which to assess the therapeutic response to phenytoin. However, in patients in whom epileptic seizures occur infrequently and irregularly and in patients taking phenytoin prophylactically (for example, after neurosurgery) it can be difficult to assess the therapeutic response. In such cases a target plasma phenytoin concentration may provide the most rational means of assessing whether or not a therapeutic response is likely to be achieved.

In all cases the signs of phenytoin toxicity may be insidious and difficult to differentiate from those of associated neurological disease. Plasma phenytoin concentration measurements may therefore help.

Is there a good relation between the plasma concentration and its therapeutic or toxic effect?

Longitudinal studies in patients with epilepsy have clearly shown improved seizure control when plasma phenytoin concentrations are increased above 40 μmol/l. Most of the patients in these studies however, had relatively severe epilepsy, and a prospective study has shown that 35% of newly diagnosed epileptic patients could have their seizures completely controlled with concentrations below 40 μmol/l. There is also evidence that even very low plasma phenytoin concentrations (5-10 μmol/l) may be associated with effective seizure control in some patients.

Nevertheless, it is generally accepted that it is more likely that optimal suppression of seizures will be achieved without toxicity when the plasma phenytoin concentration is within the range 40-80 μmol/l. The upper limit has been so defined because the risk of toxicity increases at a concentration above 80 μmol/l and is almost invariable at concentrations greater than 100 μmol/l.

Phenytoin

> The plasma phenytoin concentration range for an optimum effect in the absence of complicating factors is 40-80 μmol/l

> ### Dose dependent signs of toxicity and plasma phenytoin concentration
>
> - Nystagmus   >80 μmol/l
> - Ataxia   >120 μmol/l
> - Mental changes   >160 μmol/l

> ### Long term adverse effects of phenytoin
>
> - Gingival hyperplasia
> - Coarsening of facial features
> - Acne
> - Hirsutism
> - Folate deficiency
> - Vitamin D deficiency

Dose dependent signs of toxicity become prominent at plasma phenytoin concentrations above 80-100 μmol/l. But sometimes the signs of phenytoin toxicity are difficult to detect, especially if the patient has underlying neurological disease which might confuse the diagnosis of toxicity—for example, pre-existing cerebellar dysfunction.

Some patients may tolerate a plasma phenytoin concentration in excess of 100 μmol/l, whereas others may show signs of toxicity with a concentration less than 80 μmol/l. A plasma concentration below 80 μmol/l does not therefore exclude the possibility of toxicity, and if there are good clinical reasons for suspecting toxicity then reducing the dosage should be tried.

There is a less clear relation between plasma concentrations of phenytoin and its long term adverse effects. Many of these effects are probably related to the duration of treatment as well as to the plasma concentration.

Is phenytoin metabolised to active metabolites?

Phenytoin is metabolised to 5-(p-hydroxyphenyl)-5-phenylhydantoin (HPPH), which is clinically inactive. Less than 5% of phenytoin is excreted unchanged in the urine, so the interpretation of the plasma concentration is not complicated by the presence of pharmacologically active substances not measured by the assay.

Measurement techniques

> ### Disadvantages of measuring salivary phenytoin concentrations
>
> - Falsely high concentrations may occur in the presence of gingival hyperplasia, owing to leakage of a protein rich exudate from the inflamed gums
> - Falsely low concentrations may occur because of binding of phenytoin to cellular debris in the mouth
> - Contamination may occur if samples are collected too soon after dosing, especially with syrups
> - Salivary phenytoin concentration is about 10 times lower than the plasma concentration, and routine analytical methods are not accurate enough to measure reliably at these concentrations

Most laboratories use an enzyme linked or fluorescent immunoassay. Measurements can be made outside the laboratory using simple instruments (Seralyser, Ames) or sophisticated test strips (Acculevel, Syva). All of these methods measure the total (protein bound and unbound) plasma phenytoin concentration. In certain patients (neonates, those with chronic hepatic or renal disease, those in the third trimester of pregnancy, and those taking drugs such as sodium valproate) plasma protein binding may be reduced, and the total phenytoin concentration may greatly underestimate the concentration of unbound, pharmacologically active drug.

It is rarely possible to estimate directly the degree of impairment of binding of phenytoin to plasma proteins. An alternative approach is to measure the salivary phenytoin concentration, which correlates well with the concentration of unbound phenytoin in the plasma. However, this has several disadvantages (see box) and the routine monitoring of salivary phenytoin concentrations is therefore not recommended.

Factors affecting concentration

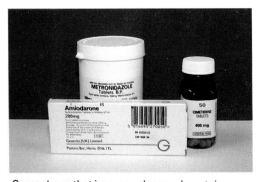

Some drugs that increase plasma phenytoin concentration by inhibiting phenytoin metabolism.

Inhibition of metabolism

Drug interactions—Cimetidine, amiodarone, allopurinol, azapropazone, chlorpromazine, imipramine, isoniazid, metronidazole, omeprazole, sulphonamides, and thioridazine all inhibit hepatic mono-oxygenase activity and may therefore cause a reduction in the rate of phenytoin metabolism, a consequent increase in plasma phenytoin concentration, and an increased risk of toxicity.

There is a complicated interaction between phenytoin and sodium valproate. Valproate displaces phenytoin from protein binding sites and thus changes the therapeutic range; it also inhibits phenytoin metabolism. This makes it difficult to interpret plasma phenytoin concentrations in patients taking valproate.

Liver disease—Acute hepatitis impairs the liver's ability to metabolise phenytoin.

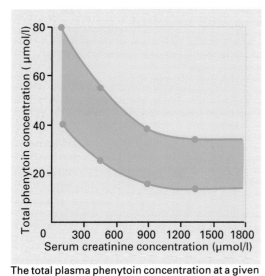

The total plasma phenytoin concentration at a given dose falls (because of reduced protein binding) as renal function worsens. Thus the therapeutic range (blue area) falls in renal failure.

Stimulation of metabolism

Drug interactions—Carbamazepine and rifampicin stimulate hepatic mono-oxygenase activity, which results in a decrease in the plasma phenytoin concentration and the consequent risk of breakthrough seizures. Folic acid increases phenytoin clearance by an unknown mechanism, thus lowering the plasma phenytoin concentration. This is important since long term treatment with phenytoin may result in a folate dependent megaloblastic anaemia. If this is treated with folic acid the plasma phenytoin concentration will be reduced, and this may result in breakthrough seizures.

Altered protein binding

Drug interactions—Aspirin and sodium valproate displace phenytoin from its binding sites on plasma albumin. The consequent increase in the fraction of unbound phenytoin in the plasma results in only a transient increase in the effect of phenytoin because it results in a proportionately increased rate of metabolism of phenytoin. The change in the proportion of unbound drug, however, alters the interpretation of the total plasma phenytoin concentration.

Hypoalbuminaemia—Chronic liver disease, the nephrotic syndrome, pregnancy, and chronic illness can all result in hypoalbuminaemia, with a consequent decrease in the number of protein binding sites for phenytoin and an increase in the unbound phenytoin concentration. As a result the plasma phenytoin concentration falls since an increase in the unbound phenytoin fraction results in an increased rate of metabolism of phenytoin.

Interpretation of plasma concentrations

Protein binding may be greatly reduced in the presence of the following:

- Hypoalbuminaemia—for example, due to severe hepatic or renal disease
- The last trimester of pregnancy, perhaps because of dilutional hypoalbuminaemia
- Renal failure, because of a reduced affinity of albumin for phenytoin
- Displacement from protein binding sites by salicylates, valproic acid, and sulphonylureas

More than 90% of plasma phenytoin is bound to albumin. Since it is the unbound fraction that is free to pass into the tissues it is this that is related to the therapeutic effect. Anything that lowers the degree of protein binding will increase the unbound fraction and therefore make it difficult to interpret the plasma phenytoin concentration, which is measured as the sum of the bound and unbound drug. In adults with no associated disease and in the absence of any displacing drug the variation in the unbound phenytoin fraction is less than twofold. In these cases measurement of the total (bound and unbound) phenytoin concentration generally provides a fairly accurate estimate of the unbound phenytoin concentration.

Since the therapeutic range for total plasma phenytoin concentrations is 40-80 μmol/l, and since about 10% of phenytoin is unbound in the plasma, a therapeutic range for free phenytoin of 4-9 μmol/l has been recommended.

Use of plasma measurements

Small changes in phenytoin dosage may cause large changes in plasma phenytoin concentration

The use of the plasma phenytoin concentration depends on whether you want to obtain adequate therapeutic concentrations to suppress fits or you want to investigate suspected toxicity.

To use the plasma concentration with a view to increasing the dosage of phenytoin it is important to wait until a steady state has been reached. It is difficult to interpret the plasma concentration if the current dosage has not been taken for a sufficient length of time for the maximum (steady state) concentration to have been reached—that is, if the plasma phenytoin concentration is still increasing with the current dosage. The unusual kinetics of phenytoin make it difficult to measure its half life and thereby predict the time at which steady state will occur. Ideally, you would measure the plasma phenytoin concentration on several successive days and when the concentration no longer increased you would know that steady state had been reached. In practice the concentration is measured after three

Phenytoin

to four weeks of continuous dosing. Given a single reliable steady state plasma concentration for a given daily dose of phenytoin, the dosage required to achieve a desired plasma concentration can be calculated by using the following simple guidelines:

- If the concentration is below 20 µmol/l an increment in daily dose of 100 mg is usually appropriate
- If the concentration is 20-60 µmol/l the daily dose should be increased by not more than 50 mg
- If the concentration is above 60 µmol/l the daily dose should be increased by only 25 mg.

If, on the other hand, you are measuring the plasma phenytoin concentration because of suspected toxicity it is not necessary to wait until steady state is reached. If the patient has symptoms or signs suggestive of toxicity and the concentration is above 80 µmol/l you can be relatively confident of the diagnosis. If clinical suspicion of toxicity is sufficiently great then a trial of reducing the dosage of phenytoin would be appropriate, even if the plasma phenytoin concentration result was below 80 µmol/l or not yet known.

Timing of measurements

The timing of plasma sampling for phenytoin is not critical

Because of the long half life of phenytoin during long term administration the diurnal fluctuation in its plasma concentration is relatively small, even when dosage is once daily. The timing of blood samples in relation to the time of dosing is therefore of little importance for correctly interpreting the plasma concentration.

The sources of the data shown in the graphs are Richens and Dunlop, *Lancet* 1975;ii:247-8 for dose *v* phenytoin concentration; Lund, *Proceedings of the Second World Conference on Clinical Pharmacology and Therapeutics* (American Society for Pharmacology and Experimental Therapeutics) 1983:40 for the relation of plasma phenytoin concentration and seizures; Kutt *et al, Archives of Neurology* 1964;11:642-8 for the relation of plasma phenytoin concentration and adverse effects; and Odar-Cederlöf, PhD thesis 1975 (Karolinska Institute, Stockholm) for plasma phenytoin concentration *v* serum creatinine concentration, and are reproduced with permission from the journals.

LITHIUM

J K Aronson, D J M Reynolds

Lithium is used in the prophylaxis of bipolar and unipolar affective disorders and in the treatment of acute mania

Serum (prepared from clotted blood) and plasma (prepared from anticoagulated blood) can be used interchangeably for other drug measurements. However, serum is usually used for measurement of lithium to avoid potential interference from lithium heparin, which is used as an anticoagulant

Monitoring serum lithium concentrations is an important part of treatment in patients with affective disorders as the drug's toxic:therapeutic ratio is very low and its pharmacokinetics vary from person to person, making accurate prediction of dosage difficult. The variation is due to differences in absorption, distribution, and elimination.

Absorption of lithium is highly variable, depending on the formulation used. The rate and extent of absorption varies between modified release and conventional formulations, but there is also variability from one modified release formulation to another.

The variations in the clearance and apparent volume of distribution of lithium result in variation in its half life from 7 hours to 41 hours.

In this chapter we apply to lithium the criteria which must be fulfilled in part or in full before measurement of its plasma concentration can be considered worth while.

Criteria for measurement

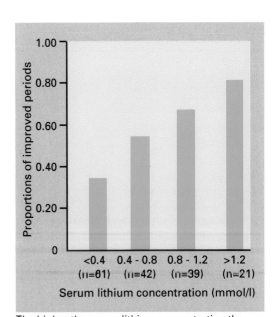

The higher the serum lithium concentration the greater the likelihood of a therapeutic response. In acute mania the chance of a therapeutic response continued to improve up to relatively high serum concentrations.

Is there difficulty in interpreting clinical evidence of the therapeutic or toxic effects?

Although it may be possible to achieve a steady state serum lithium concentration within the therapeutic range relatively rapidly (for example, by giving a loading dose), the onset of a detectable therapeutic action in patients with acute mania may be delayed for up to two weeks.

Even when a therapeutic effect has occurred it may be difficult to know whether the effect is optimal and whether it is attributable to the drug or to spontaneous remission. Furthermore, assessment of the extent to which lithium is contributing to a change in mood may be difficult in patients taking other mood altering drugs, as is commonly the case.

Furthermore, lithium is used for prophylaxis in patients with recurrent unipolar and bipolar affective illnesses. In such cases although a relapse may be evidence of a lack of therapeutic effect, you cannot be sure that the prophylactic dose is optimal in patients who remain in remission. In addition, such patients may well experience mild adverse effects of lithium, which occur commonly with therapeutic dosages. It may therefore be difficult to find a dosage that is effective and does not cause adverse effects.

Is there a good relation between the serum concentration and its therapeutic or toxic effects?

Because serum lithium concentrations vary quite widely between doses it is important that they are measured at a standard time. We will call this measurement the standard serum lithium concentration.

Interpretation of the results of studies of the relation between serum concentrations of lithium and its therapeutic effect has been made difficult by the fact that in many such studies measurement of serum lithium concentration has not been made at the same standard time after the previous dose. Despite this there is some evidence that a therapeutic effect is most likely to be achieved in patients with acute mania if the standard serum lithium concentration is above 0·8 mmol/l. There is also evidence

Lithium

> The therapeutic range for steady state standard serum lithium concentrations in the treatment of acute mania is 0·8-1·2 mmol/l

> The therapeutic steady state serum concentration range for lithium in the prophylaxis of unipolar and bipolar affective illness is 0·4-0·8 mmol/l

Acute toxic effects
- Gastrointestinal symptoms—nausea, vomiting, diarrhoea
- Neuromuscular disorders—muscle weakness and fasciculation
- Central nervous system effects—confusion, ataxia, dysarthria, convulsions
- Cardiac arrhythmias
- Renal impairment

Long term adverse effects independent of serum lithium concentration
- Thirst and polyuria
- Tremor
- Weight gain (partly due to water retention, sometimes with oedema)
- Diarrhoea
- Hypothyroidism

that there is little benefit to be gained by increasing the concentration above 1·2 mmol/l and that the risk of adverse effects increases considerably above this concentration. Thus a reasonable therapeutic range for steady state standard serum lithium concentrations in patients with acute mania is 0·8-1·2 mmol/l.

The evidence for a relation between the steady state standard concentration and a therapeutic effect in the prophylaxis of unipolar and bipolar affective illness is even less clear. The available evidence suggests that a lower range of concentrations is associated with a therapeutic effect compared with that for acute mania. It is common practice to maintain concentrations in the range 0·4-0·8 mmol/l, though there is little firm evidence to suggest that an optimal therapeutic effect will thus be obtained. It is likely, however, that by keeping the concentration below 0·8 mmol/l the risk of adverse effects will be reduced, though not eliminated.

Long term remissions can, however, occur in patients with serum lithium concentrations below 0·4 mmol/l and this is not seen as a reason for withdrawing treatment (in contrast to digoxin—see p 35). Conversely, in some patients a therapeutic effect in prophylaxis is achieved only by giving dosages associated with serum concentrations above 0·8 mmol/l.

It is generally agreed that the risk of lithium toxicity increases considerably when the steady state standard serum lithium concentration exceeds 1·4 mmol/l. The adverse effects that occur during acute toxicity are listed in the box. Note that lithium induced renal impairment leads to worsened toxicity through retention of lithium.

In contrast it is not clear what the relation is between the steady state standard serum lithium concentration and the risk of adverse effects during long term treatment when the concentration is below 1·4 mmol/l. For example, it has been reported that only 10% of patients with serum concentrations within the range 0·4-1·3 mmol/l escape adverse effects. On the other hand, there is evidence that the frequency and severity of adverse effects may be reduced when serum concentrations are reduced from 0·9 mmol/l to 0·7 mmol/l. It should be noted, however, that this conclusion was based on retrospective comparisons of patients studied at different times.

The major long term adverse effects encountered by patients with serum concentrations in the therapeutic range are listed in the box. It is no longer thought that long term treatment with lithium is associated with renal damage. This is in contrast to the acute nephrotoxic effect that may occur when lithium concentrations exceed the therapeutic range.

Measurement techniques

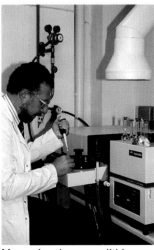

Measuring the serum lithium concentration by flame emission photometry.

Lithium concentrations are measured by either flame emission photometry or atomic absorption spectrophotometry.

When collecting samples for measurement it is better to use clotted blood, from which serum can be separated, rather than anticoagulated blood. This is to avoid possible confusion in cases in which lithium heparin is used as an anticoagulant. Serum should be separated as quickly as possible, since there is movement of lithium into erythrocytes after that time. Although it has been recommended that serum is best separated within an hour of sampling, it is not clear how important that is, and some have recommended that it is acceptable to leave samples for longer (for example, up to 24 h) before separation. Perhaps the best advice is to try to standardise the time of separation to within a few hours on all occasions.

Factors affecting the concentration

Factors that cause increased serum lithium concentrations

- Reduced glomerular filtration rate
- Sodium depletion
- Drugs:
  Diuretics (principally thiazides)
  Non-steroidal anti-inflammatory drugs
  (which may also reduce the
  glomerular filtration rate)
- Vomiting and diarrhoea
- Fever

As absorption of lithium from different oral formulations is variable different steady state serum concentrations may result if the formulation is changed.

Since lithium is eliminated from the body almost completely by renal excretion, factors that impair its excretion will cause increased serum concentrations. These factors are listed in the box.

Conversely, an increase in glomerular filtration rate, as occurs in the second half of pregnancy, will cause an increased rate of lithium excretion. (Note, however, that lithium is teratogenic and should not be given at least during the first trimester of pregnancy.)

Factors affecting interpretation

Drugs that may potentiate the toxic effects of lithium

- Neuroleptics:
  Haloperidol
- Antidepressants:
  Fluoxetine
- Calcium antagonists:
  Diltiazem
  Verapamil
- Anticonvulsants:
  Carbamazepine
  Phenytoin

The actions of lithium may be enhanced by concurrent treatment with other drugs (see box) and by electroconvulsive therapy. It is not clear how to interpret the serum lithium concentrations in these circumstances. In general you should use the lowest dosages of neuroleptics possible if lithium is also to be used, and some psychiatrists withdraw lithium two or three days before electroconvulsive therapy.

Use of serum measurements

Case history: effects of sodium depletion

A 68 year old man developed a flu-like illness, with fever and diarrhoea. He continued to take lithium and within a few days became weak and drowsy, dysarthric, and ataxic. His serum lithium concentration was 3·1 mmol/l and he had acute renal failure. Lithium was withdrawn and he was rehydrated. Serial serum lithium concentration measurements over the next 24 hours showed that his serum lithium concentration was not falling quickly enough, and since he remained unwell he underwent dialysis, with a good result.

Conclusion

This case illustrates the need to warn patients to reduce the dosage of lithium and to seek medical advice if they develop fever or diarrhoea, or both. It also highlights the problems that can arise if there is impaired renal function.

It is possible to establish a dosage regimen of lithium in prophylaxis by giving 0·15-0·20 mmol/kg/day (that is, 10-14 mmol/day in a 70 kg patient, or about 400-600 mg/day of lithium carbonate) and measuring the serum lithium concentration no less than a week later, when a steady state can be assumed to have been reached. The dosage can then be adjusted in proportion to the desired target steady state concentration, as described below. The corresponding starting dosage in patients with acute mania would be 0·3-0·4 mmol/kg/day (about 25 mmol/day for a 70 kg patient, or about 1 g/day of lithium carbonate). The total dosage should be given in divided doses throughout the day.

It is possible to plan a dosage regimen in an individual patient more rationally by using the serum lithium concentration measured one or more times during initial treatment. The simplest method described[1] entails giving a test dose of lithium carbonate (1·2 g) followed by measurement of the serum concentration 24 hours later. The serum concentration is then put into an equation that predicts the steady state serum concentration that would result from a daily maintenance dose of 1·8 g. As the maintenance dose is directly proportional to the steady state concentration this dose can be scaled down to achieve the target steady state concentration. For example, if a daily maintenance dosage of 1·8 g a day produced a steady state concentration of 1·2 mmol/l a dosage of 1·2 g would result in a concentration of about 0·8 mmol/l.

Lithium

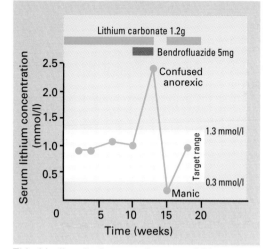

Thiazide diuretics increase the serum lithium concentration.

We believe that there is little merit in regularly checking serum lithium concentrations, and such checks may be reserved for times when you suspect that the patient's condition has changed in some way that would affect the concentration (see boxes on p 19). Because of this it is important to warn the patient to seek advice when changes of this kind occur. However, others recommend that serum lithium concentrations should be measured at least every three months, regardless of whether there is an indication for measurement. In our view such measurement is not a substitute for regularly reviewing the patient's clinical condition and reminding patients of the risk factors associated with toxicity.

Case history: interaction with thiazide diuretics

A 58 year old woman had been well stabilised on lithium with serum lithium concentrations varying from 0·5 to 0·8 mmol/l.
She developed peripheral oedema and was treated with bendrofluazide.
She was admitted to hospital a week later with delirium. Her serum lithium concentration was 2·5 mmol/l. The lithium and diuretic were withdrawn and 36 hours later she was well. Lithium was restarted in the same dosage without subsequent problems. Her oedema was attributed to lithium and was treated satisfactorily with amiloride.

Conclusion
This case illustrates an interaction of lithium and a thiazide diuretic.

It is also important to measure the serum lithium concentration when patients develop troublesome adverse effects, when the concentration may be used as a guide to reductions in dosage.

The serum lithium concentration may also be used to check patient compliance.

Timing of measurements

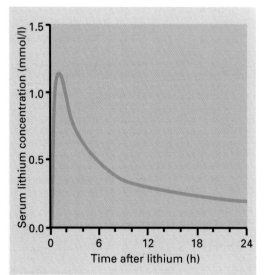

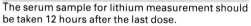

The serum sample for lithium measurement should be taken 12 hours after the last dose.

Two factors affect the timing of blood samples in patients taking lithium. Firstly, the considerable variation in the plasma lithium concentration during a single interval between dosages has led to the concept of a standardised time of sampling—namely, at 12 hours after the previous dose. Secondly, there is a diurnal variation in the handling of lithium by the body, and the half life of lithium is longer during the night than during the day. Although this has implications for the way in which a dose taken twice daily might be split, current regimens do not take diurnal variation into account.

It is therefore important when monitoring therapy to try to take the blood sample as close as possible to 12 hours after the last dose, and preferably always at the same time of day. This is possible in patients who are seen in the morning, having taken their last dose the previous night. It raises practical problems, however, in patients who are seen in the afternoon. These problems can be ameliorated to some extent if patients are given modified release formulations to take twice a day, since these formulations tend to even out the diurnal variations in serum concentrations.

1 Perry PJ, Alexander B, Prince RA, Dunner FJ. The utility of a single-point dosing protocol for predicting steady-state lithium levels. *Br J Psychiatry* 1986;**148**:401-5.

The sources of the data shown in the graphs are Stokes *et al*, *Arch Gen Psychiatry* 1976;**33**:1080-4 for improved periods with serum lithium concentrations; Brodie, *Medicine International* 1988;**59**:2435-9 for the effect of bendrofluazide; and Amdisen, *Danish Med Bull* 1975;**22**:227 for lithium concentration *v* time, and are reproduced with permission of the journals.

THEOPHYLLINE

J K Aronson, M Hardman, D J M Reynolds

Theophylline is a xanthine that is used in the treatment of asthma, both for long term prophylaxis and for acute severe attacks

It is not possible to establish a single dosage regimen for theophylline or its derivatives (for example, aminophylline) that will suit all patients because the metabolism of theophylline varies greatly from person to person. This variation is reflected in its elimination half life, which varies from four hours in healthy adult smokers to about 25 hours in patients with hepatic cirrhosis.

Several of the factors responsible for the variation (age, smoking habits, body weight, diet, concomitant illness, and drug interactions) can be considered when estimating the most appropriate dosage regimen. But the therapeutic:toxic ratio for theophylline is very small, and only by measuring the plasma theophylline concentration can the dosage be tailored for individual patients.

In this chapter we apply to theophylline the criteria that must be fulfilled in part or in full before the measurement of its plasma concentration can be considered worth while.

Criteria for measurement

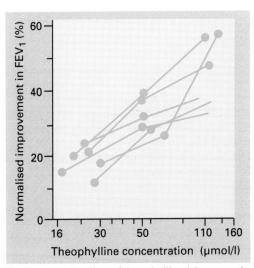

The therapeutic effect of theophylline (shown as the change in FEV$_1$) increased with increasing plasma concentration in six patients with asthma.

The plasma theophylline concentration range for an optimum effect in the absence of complicating factors is 55-110 μmol/l

Is there difficulty in interpreting clinical evidence of the therapeutic or toxic effects?

There is a relation between the dose of theophylline and the reduction in airways resistance achieved. The drug's chief therapeutic effect, however, is the relief of bronchoconstriction, which is only one of the three factors that cause airways obstruction in asthma, the other two being mucosal oedema and mucus plugging of the airways. Thus in asthmatic patients a change in FEV$_1$, which reflects all three factors, is an unreliable guide to theophylline dosing, and monitoring of plasma concentrations is essential in order to optimise treatment.

Many patients experience gastrointestinal symptoms when their plasma concentration is within the therapeutic range, but minor adverse effects do not always precede major ones. Several of the adverse effects (nervousness, tachycardia, arrhythmias, and cardiorespiratory arrest) can be features of an acute attack of asthma, and it may be impossible to distinguish between features of the underlying disease and those attributable to theophylline toxicity without measuring the plasma theophylline concentration.

Is there a good relation between the plasma concentration and its therapeutic or toxic effects?

In experimental studies there is a linear relation between changes in forced expiratory volume in the first second (FEV$_1$) and the logarithm of the plasma theophylline concentration over the range 17-110 μmol/l. Improvement in FEV$_1$ is often only slight with concentrations less than 55 μmol/l, and clinical evidence suggests that 55 μmol/l may be considered as the lower limit of the therapeutic range. The upper limit is generally accepted as 110 μmol/l, which is the concentration at which agitation and tachycardia usually become apparent.

Minor adverse effects, such as nausea, insomnia, nervousness, and headache, are common if the plasma theophylline concentration is rapidly increased above 55 μmol/l. Most patients will tolerate the drug better if the dose is gradually increased to attain maintenance plasma concentrations in the middle or upper part of the therapeutic range. About 5% of patients

Theophylline

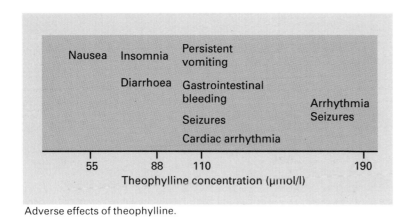

Adverse effects of theophylline.

develop unacceptable nausea and diarrhoea at plasma concentrations below 80 µmol/l. Serious adverse effects—persistent vomiting, gastrointestinal bleeding, seizures, cardiac arrhythmias, and cardiorespiratory arrest—often occur at concentrations above 110 µmol/l. Plasma concentrations above 190 µmol/l are invariably associated with a high risk of dangerous cardiac arrhythmias.

Is theophylline metabolised to active metabolites?

Theophylline is metabolised in the liver to 1,3-dimethyluric acid and, by N-methylation of both theophylline and 1,3-dimethyluric acid, to 1-methyluric acid and 3-methylxanthine. The metabolites are excreted through the kidney, along with about 10% of the unchanged drug. The 3-methylxanthine metabolite is not as active as theophylline, so the presence of active metabolites does not create a problem in interpreting the plasma theophylline concentration.

Measurement techniques

> Theophylline can be detected rapidly by immunoassay

Most laboratories use an enzyme linked or fluorescent immunoassay. A paper test strip (Acculevel, Syva, Maidenhead), to which a capillary blood sample is applied, provides a theophylline assay within 30 minutes, but this method is expensive and is not widely used in the United Kingdom.

Factors affecting concentration

Factors that affect the plasma theophylline concentration

Factors that increase concentration

Formulation: Elixirs *v* modified release formulations

Age: Premature babies; neonates; elderly people

Weight: Obesity

Diet: High carbohydrate; low protein; dietary methylxanthines

Diseases: Chronic obstructive airways disease; pneumonia; hepatic cirrhosis; heart failure

Drugs: Allopurinol; cimetidine; macrolide antibiotics (such as erythromycin); oral contraceptives; viloxazine

Factors that reduce concentration

Age: Children

Diet: Low carbohydrate; high protein; charcoal cooked meats

Drugs: Carbamazepine; phenobarbitone; phenytoin; rifampicin; sulphinpyrazone

Smoking

Certain factors can increase or decrease the plasma theophylline concentration. Some (for example, the patient's age and body weight, and concurrent diseases) are beyond the prescriber's control but should be borne in mind when choosing dosage regimens. Others are under the prescriber's control—for example, the plasma concentration during treatment can be manipulated by choosing different formulations (elixirs, conventional formulations, and modified release formulations). Furthermore, it is important to know about drug interactions which may alter the plasma theophylline concentration. These are of two types: those in which theophylline metabolism is inhibited and its plasma concentration increased, and those in which its metabolism is stimulated and its plasma concentration reduced (see box).

Use of plasma measurements

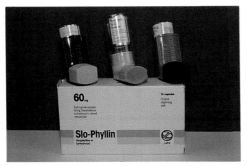

Some drugs used in the treatment of asthma.

Prophylaxis

In patients with recurrent severe attacks of asthma theophylline is often added to the regimen if combinations of inhaled β₂ adrenoceptor agonists (such as salbutamol) and a corticosteroid are inadequate. It is important to ensure that the patient is receiving an adequate dosage of theophylline to provide optimum protection against further acute attacks of asthma. The patient's respiratory function test results during an episode of remission cannot, however, be used to assess the therapeutic response to theophylline. This can be achieved only by measuring the plasma theophylline concentration and by adjusting the dosage so that the concentration is within the therapeutic range. This assumes that the patient does not experience any adverse effects of theophylline.

Case history: drug interaction

A 72 year old man with longstanding obstructive airways disease treated with modified release aminophylline had an acute infective exacerbation of his symptoms. He was given erythromycin by his general practitioner and after a week his breathing was much improved. However, two days later he developed severe nausea and vomiting and was admitted to hospital after suffering a small haematemesis. The plasma theophylline concentration on admission was 120 μmol/l. Aminophylline and erythromycin were withdrawn and his condition improved. A few days later his breathing had worsened, with an associated fall in FEV_1, and aminophylline was restarted in his usual maintenance dosage. The plasma theophylline concentration two weeks later was 90 μmol/l.

Conclusion

There was an interaction between erythromycin and theophylline in this patient. A reduction in the maintenance dosage of theophylline of the order of 25% is required if macrolide antibiotics are continued for more than five days.

Case history: problems caused by previous theophylline

A 19 year old woman was admitted to hospital with a severe attack of acute asthma. No information was available on her current drug therapy, and she was too unwell to volunteer the information. Her condition worsened despite nebulised salbutamol and ipratropium, so an intravenous infusion of aminophylline 500 mg was given over 30 minutes. Towards the end of the infusion she had a cardiac arrest, was successfully resuscitated, and was transferred to the intensive therapy unit. The plasma theophylline concentration three hours after the end of the infusion was 245 μmol/l. It subsequently transpired that she had been taking oral theophylline daily for some years and indeed had increased the dose during the two days before admission because of worsening asthma.

Conclusion

This case illustrates the danger of giving intravenous theophylline to patients who are already taking oral theophylline.

Routine therapy

Patients taking theophylline for chronic reversible airways obstruction whose condition is not adequately controlled may require an increased dosage. Measuring the plasma concentration allows the clinician to adjust the dosage without risking the toxic effects, which in most cases can be predicted from the plasma concentration. For example, if the patient has a plasma theophylline concentration below 55 μmol/l the dosage can be safely increased, whereas if the concentration is above 110 μmol/l the risk of toxicity with an increase in dosage is much greater. Knowing the plasma concentration would allow the most appropriate change in dosage to be made.

The plasma concentration is linearly related to dosage, and increases in dosage can be calculated on that basis. For example, in a patient taking 500 mg of aminophylline a day with a steady state plasma theophylline concentration of 60 μmol/l, increasing the total daily dose of aminophylline to 750 mg would be expected to increase the steady state theophylline concentration to 90 μmol/l.

In acute asthma a knowledge of the plasma theophylline concentration is useful for two reasons. Firstly, if it is measured before theophylline is given it reduces the risk of theophylline toxicity, which can arise if a patient already taking the drug is given an intravenous loading dose. It is therefore important to ask patients whether they have been taking theophylline before coming into hospital. Remember that certain over the counter remedies (for example, Dodo tablets) contain theophylline. Secondly, if the patient has not responded to intravenous theophylline the rate of infusion can be increased to ensure that the optimal dosage is being administered without unnecessarily risking severe toxicity.

Toxicity

Measuring the plasma theophylline concentration will help to confirm a diagnosis of theophylline toxicity. In a case of theophylline overdose measuring the plasma concentration will help to assess the prognosis, plan the treatment, and assess the response to treatment.

Timing of measurements

Intravenous infusion—Take the sample after 4-6 hours of infusion, having stopped the infusion for 15 minutes

Oral administration—Take the sample 8-12 hours after the last dose. For sequential monitoring take samples at the same time each day

Intravenous infusion

During intravenous infusion a sample for measurement of plasma theophylline concentration may be taken at any time if theophylline toxicity is suspected. If there are no adverse effects a sample should be taken four to six hours after the start of the infusion, and the infusion should be stopped for 15 minutes before a sample is taken so that the plasma concentration reflects the total body concentration; otherwise the plasma theophylline concentration may be significantly higher because of the diffusion gradient from the plasma to the tissues.

Theophylline

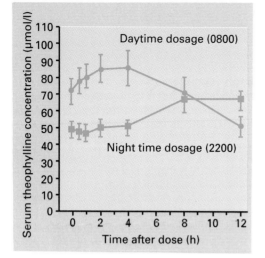

The plasma concentration profile during the 12 hours after a dose of theophylline depends on the time of day the drug was taken. Plasma concentrations are higher after daytime administration. (Data from 13 asthmatic children who took a modified release formulation.)

Oral theophylline

In patients taking oral theophylline ideally a "trough" (minimum steady state) plasma concentration should be measured. The time at which the "peak" plasma concentration occurs varies from 15 minutes after the dose (for elixirs) to two hours (for ordinary formulations) and four to six hours (for modified release formulations). This strictly limits the period during which the sample should be taken. As there is a circadian rhythm of theophylline metabolism, resulting in higher trough concentrations in the morning than later in the day, repeat samples for measurement of the trough concentration should be taken at the same time of day as previous samples to allow direct comparison of the results.

Given all these considerations the most practical strategy for routine monitoring is to tell the patient to take the morning dose on wakening and to measure the plasma theophylline concentration during the afternoon. Modified release formulations may be taken at night, with measurement of the plasma concentration the next morning.

The sources of the data presented in the graphs are: Mitenko and Ogilvie, *N Engl J Med* 1973;**289**:600-3 for the therapeutic effect of theophylline; and Smolensky *et al*, *J Asthma* 1987;**24**: 90-134 for theophylline concentration *v* time after dose. The data are reproduced with permission of the journals.

AMINOGLYCOSIDE ANTIBIOTICS

J K Aronson, D J M Reynolds

Aminoglycoside antibiotics (including amikacin, gentamicin, kanamycin, tobramycin, and netilmicin) are used in the treatment of serious systemic infections such as infective endocarditis and Gram negative septicaemia. Streptomycin is used in the treatment of tuberculosis

Monitoring the serum concentrations of aminoglycoside antibiotics is an important part of treatment as their toxic:therapeutic ratio is very low. In addition, the pharmacokinetics of aminoglycosides vary considerably from person to person, making accurate prediction of initial dosage difficult. The sources of this variation are differences in renal function and tissue distribution.

The aminoglycosides are almost completely cleared unchanged from the body by renal excretion; clearance is therefore subject to variation when renal function varies. This is important for two reasons. Firstly, renal function is often impaired in patients with severe sepsis, in whom aminoglycosides are often indicated; furthermore, as the infection resolves improvement in renal function may further alter the pharmacokinetics of the antibiotic. Secondly, the aminoglycosides are themselves nephrotoxic and may therefore impair their own disposition. If this happens a vicious cycle of renal impairment with worsening toxicity may arise. Although the renal toxicity is usually reversible, accumulation of the aminoglycoside may lead to ototoxicity, which may be irreversible.

The distribution of the aminoglycosides to the tissues varies among patients because of a wide range of factors, including age, fever, body weight, anaemia, drug interactions, and overall severity of illness.

The variations in the clearance and apparent volume of distribution of gentamicin result in variation in its initial half life from 0·4 h to 7·6 h in patients with normal renal function.

In this chapter we apply to aminoglycosides the criteria which must be fulfilled in part or in full before the measurement of their plasma concentrations can be considered worth while.

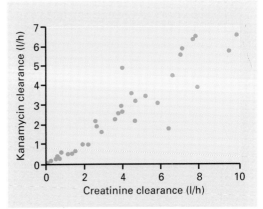

The clearance of aminoglycoside antibiotics from the body falls as renal function falls.

Criteria for measurement

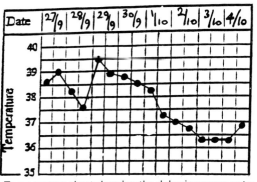

Temperature chart showing the delay in response to an antibiotic.

Is there difficulty in interpreting clinical evidence of the therapeutic or toxic effects?

Therapeutic responses to aminoglycosides may take several days to become clinically apparent. It is therefore important during the early phases of treatment to know that you are giving a dose which is likely to have an eventual therapeutic effect. To do this you need to measure the serum concentration, as there is a poor relation between dose and serum concentration but a good relation between serum concentration and the therapeutic effect. Furthermore, even when a therapeutic response starts to occur it can be difficult to know whether it is optimal. Again, measurement of the concentration will help.

As far as renal toxicity is concerned, it is impossible to distinguish clinically between renal impairment secondary to the illness and that secondary to a toxic effect of the aminoglycosides. However, diagnosing the cause of renal impairment is a secondary consideration, and measurement of the serum aminoglycoside concentration is used to prevent toxicity rather than to diagnose drug induced renal toxicity.

As we describe below, the problem of ototoxicity is more complicated.

Aminoglycoside antibiotics

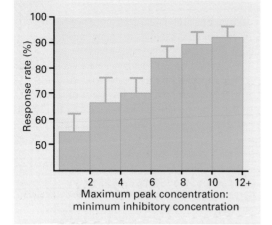

The higher the serum gentamicin concentration in relation to the in vitro minimum inhibitory concentration (MIC), the greater the therapeutic effect.

Minimum peak concentrations for a therapeutic response

Gentamicin, tobramycin, netilmicin	5 μg/ml
Amikacin, kanamycin	20 μg/ml

Maximum peak concentrations to avoid toxicity

Gentamicin, tobramycin, netilmicin	10 μg/ml
Amikacin, kanamycin	30 μg/ml

Maximum trough concentrations to avoid toxixity

Gentamicin, tobramycin, netilmicin	2 μg/ml
Amikacin, kanamycin	10 μg/ml

Is there a good relation between the serum concentration and therapeutic or toxic effects?

The therapeutic effect of an antibacterial drug conventionally is assessed by measuring the minimum inhibitory concentration of the drug for the infective organism in vitro. The effective serum concentration is then considered to be achieved when it is higher than the in vitro minimum inhibitory concentration. However, this does not guarantee that an effective tissue concentration will be achieved, since penetration of the drug to the affected tissue will vary among patients and with the infection. This may be affected by factors such as tissue blood flow and host defence mechanisms, including numbers and function of white cells.

Because of these difficulties, recommended target serum concentrations for a therapeutic effect have been based on the results of clinical studies, which have shown that a serum concentration of gentamicin of 5 μg/ml or more 15 minutes after the end of an intravenous infusion or 1 hour after an intravenous bolus or an intramuscular injection should be achieved. The corresponding values for other aminoglycosides are given in the box. Factors that can alter this concentration are discussed below.

There is some debate about the relation between serum concentrations of aminoglycosides and their nephrotoxic and ototoxic effects (see below). For practical purposes, however, it is generally accepted that the risks of adverse effects will be reduced if peak serum concentrations of gentamicin are below 10 μg/ml and if trough concentrations (that is, just before the next dose) are below 2 μg/ml. (See box for other aminoglycosides.)

With increasing interest in the use of once a day regimens of high doses of some aminoglycosides it will be necessary to redefine the relations between serum concentrations and the therapeutic and toxic effects of these drugs. There is currently little information on this and we shall not deal with it further.

Measurement techniques

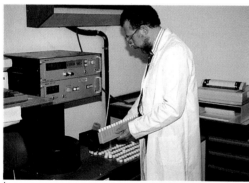

Immunoassay is the usual method for measuring aminoglycosides concentrations.

As heparin may interfere with measurement of aminoglycoside concentrations serum samples should be used.

Although the serum concentrations of aminoglycosides can be measured by using their ability to inhibit the growth of bacteria in vitro, bioassays of this kind take too long to be of maximum practical value. For this reason it is now customary to use immunoassay. It is also possible to use high performance liquid chromatography, but this is generally reserved for research purposes.

Factors affecting the serum concentration

The main factor that affects serum aminoglycoside concentrations at a given dose is renal impairment. For this reason extra care should be taken in elderly patients.

Since the aminoglycosides are excreted almost exclusively by the kidneys renal function is the main factor affecting serum glycoside concentrations. Dosages of gentamicin should therefore be reduced in patients with renal impairment, using the serum concentration as a guide. Since elderly people may have impaired renal function, age is also an important factor.

There have been reports that frusemide may increase plasma gentamicin concentrations by impairing its renal excretion. However, the interaction of the drugs is complicated by the fact that both frusemide and the aminoglycosides have direct ototoxic effects. This combination is therefore better avoided, and if a loop diuretic is required in a patient also receiving an aminoglycoside then bumetanide, which is less ototoxic than frusemide, is to be preferred.

Factors affecting interpretation

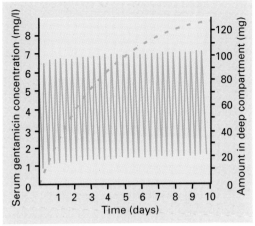

Tissue accumulation of aminoglycoside antibiotics increases during repeated administration over several days, even though the serum concentrations do not increase during that time.

The relation between the serum aminoglycoside concentration and its toxic effects changes with duration of treatment. This is because as treatment proceeds aminoglycosides tend to accumulate in the tissues without there being at the same time a comparable increase in the peak and trough serum concentrations. This means that a serum concentration that was not associated with toxic effects during the first few days of treatment can be associated with toxic effects during longer term treatment. The risk of toxicity begins to increase after about a week of continuous treatment.

The most important consequence of this change in the relation between serum and tissue concentrations is that with increasing duration of treatment there is an increased risk of ototoxicity and nephrotoxicity. Special care should therefore be taken in any patient in whom treatment may need to be continued for more than one week. Important indications for this category include infections due to Gram negative organisms; organisms, such as *Enterococcus faecalis*, causing infective endocarditis; osteomyelitis; and infections of vascular grafts. In these patients it is wise, if possible, to determine baseline auditory and vestibular function before treatment and to reassess after one week and then at weekly intervals. It may also be advisable in some circumstances to use netilmicin, which is thought to be less ototoxic than other aminoglycosides.

When the aminoglycosides are used in combination with other antibiotics for the treatment of infections with enterococci and *viridans* streptococci there may be synergy, the effective peak serum concentrations may be lower than usual (3-5 μg/ml).

Use of serum measurements

Case history: high peak/acceptable trough

A 55 year old man with a serum creatinine concentration of 110 μmol/l was given gentamicin and benzylpenicillin for infective endocarditis due to *viridans* streptococci. After a loading dose of 120 mg and two maintenance doses of 80 mg at eight hourly intervals his peak gentamicin concentration was 18 μg/ml and his trough concentration 1·2 μg/ml. The dosing interval in this case was thus equal to about four half lives (18-9, 9-4·5, 4·5-2·25, and 2·25-1·125 μg/ml). The maintenance dose was halved to 40 mg, and the peak concentration fell to 9 μg/ml. The dosage interval was reduced by 25% to six hours (three half lives), and this achieved approximately the same trough concentration as before.

Conclusion
Safe treatment was achieved by reducing the total daily dose from 240 mg to 160 mg and by using a different dosage interval.

Patients with normal renal function usually start treatment with a loading dose (say 120 mg intravenously or intramuscularly) and then continue with a maintenance dosage of about 80 mg three times a day in the first instance. After 24 hours take two blood samples, one just before giving the next dose to measure the trough concentration, and the other soon after the next dose to measure the peak concentration. Blood samples should not be taken through lines through which the drug has been given.

Subsequent dosages should be based on both the peak and trough concentrations. Note that a dosage adjustment aimed at altering the peak concentration will also alter the trough concentration and it is therefore often necessary to alter both the total dose given and the frequency of administration.

Case history: ototoxicity during long term treatment

A 60 year old man with mild mitral regurgitation developed an influenza-like illness, and *Enterococcus faecalis* was grown from his blood. He was given ampicillin and gentamicin intravenously. The loading dose of gentamicin was 120 mg and the maintenance dose 80 mg eight hourly. His peak and trough serum concentrations during steady state treatment were always satisfactory. After two weeks his mitral regurgitation was worse, so gentamicin was given for a further three weeks. His peak and trough concentrations continued to be acceptable. At the end of this time his mitral regurgitation had improved and gentamicin was stopped. However, he was unsteady on his feet, and formal testing showed impaired auditory and vestibular function. Although some of this impairment reversed, he was left with a slight residual disability.

Conclusion
This case illustrates that adverse effects of the aminoglycosides can occur during long term treatment despite satisfactory serum concentrations throughout the period of treatment.

Case history: high peak/high trough

A 78 year old woman with a serum creatinine concentration of 160 μmol/l was admitted with septicaemia caused by *Escherichia coli* secondary to a urinary tract infection. She was given ampicillin and gentamicin intravenously. Because of her increased creatinine concentration the initial loading dose of gentamicin was 80 mg, and this was followed by maintenance doses of 60 mg at intervals of eight hours. Despite this reduction in dosage her peak serum gentamicin concentration two days later was 16 μg/ml and the trough concentration was 8 μg/ml. The dosing interval in this case was thus equal to one half-life (16-8 μg/ml). The next dose was therefore delayed until the serum concentration had fallen to 2 μg/ml (that is, two half lives or 16 hours). At this stage 2/16 of the original body load was still present.

Conclusion
The target concentration of 8 μg/ml was achieved by giving about 6/16 of the original maintenance dose (that is, 25 mg). The subsequent dosage interval was 16 hours (two half lives), and this achieved approximately the same trough concentration of 2 μg/ml.

Timing of measurements

Timing of measurements

Intravenous infusion

- Peak—15 mins after the end of the infusion
- Trough—just before the next dose

Intramuscular or bolus intravenous dose

- Peak—1 hour after the dose
- Trough—just before the next dose

Blood samples for serum aminoglycoside measurements are generally taken immediately before a dose (the trough concentration) and soon after the next dose (the peak concentration). Although this is the order in which the samples are taken, it is generally assumed for dosage calculations that the trough concentration is that measured after the peak rather than before it.

The time of sampling for the peak concentration depends on the route of administration. If the aminoglycoside is given by intravenous infusion samples should be taken 15 minutes after the end of the infusion. If the dose is given by intravenous bolus or intramuscularly they should be taken one hour after the injection.

The sources of data presented in the graphs are: B M Orme and R E Cutler, *Clin Pharmacol Ther* 1969; 10:543-50 for creatinine clearance *v* kanamycin clearance; R D Moore, P S Lietman, and C R Smith, *J Infect Dis* 1987;155:93-9 for relationship between peak concentration: MIC and rate of response; and M Wenk, S Vozeh, and F Follath, *Clin Pharmacokinetics* 1984; 9:475-92 for tissue accumulation of aminoglycosides. The data are reproduced with permission of the journals.

CYCLOSPORIN

D J M Reynolds, J K Aronson

Cyclosporin is primarily used to prevent the rejection of transplanted organs. However, it has also been used in a wide range of other conditions, including psoriasis, rheumatoid arthritis, and asthma

Monitoring whole blood concentrations of cyclosporin is an important part of treatment since its toxic:therapeutic ratio is very low. Also, the variable pharmacokinetics of cyclosporin among patients make accurate prediction of the initial dosage difficult. This variability results from differences in the drug's absorption, distribution, and clearance.

Cyclosporin is fat soluble and some of the variability in its disposition may result from distribution into body fat. In addition, its apparent volume of distribution may be altered in patients with liver or renal disease.

Another important aspect in its distribution is that it is highly bound to erythrocytes and plasma lipoproteins. At low blood concentrations (below 80 nmol/l (100 ng/ml)) and when the packed cell volume is low (for example, in patients with kidney failure) the contribution of the plasma bound fraction becomes more important to the disposition of the drug.

Cyclosporin is metabolised in the liver and its clearance may therefore be reduced in patients with liver disease. Both cyclosporin and its metabolites are excreted in bile and little cyclosporin appears in the urine. Thus renal impairment does not alter the elimination of cyclosporin.

Measurement techniques

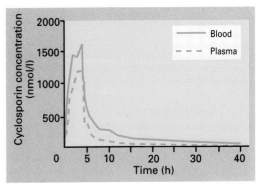

Type of sample: the concentrations during and after a 4 hour infusion in the same patient were higher when measured by radioimmunoassay in whole blood than in plasma.

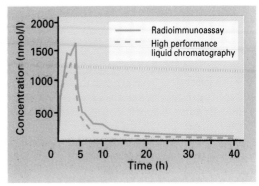

Type of assay: the concentrations during and after a 4 hour infusion in the same patient were higher when measured by radioimmunoassay than by high performance liquid chromatography.

The method of measuring the blood cyclosporin concentration is crucial to its use in monitoring treatment.

Blood cyclosporin concentration is determined by two factors: the element of the blood used for the assay (plasma, serum, or whole blood) and the type of assay.

Type of sample

The distribution of cyclosporin into erythrocytes is temperature dependent. The drug tends to bind to erythrocyte membranes after sampling, particularly if the sample is allowed to cool. For this reason some investigators separate the plasma or serum from whole blood samples at 37°C and reheat to 37°C samples which have been allowed to cool. Others prefer to separate all plasma and serum samples at 4°C. An alternative method is to measure the concentration in whole blood, in which case temperature is irrelevant.

Ethylenediamine tetraacetic acid (EDTA) should be used as an anticoagulant and blood should not be drawn through plastic cannulas through which cyclosporin has previously been given.

Type of assay

Two main assay techniques are available: radioimmunoassay and high performance liquid chromatography.

Early radioimmunoassays used non-specific antibodies, which cross reacted with metabolites of cyclosporin. More recently, however, antibodies (both monoclonal and polyclonal) specific for cyclosporin have been developed, and these may yield more reproducible results. Indeed, the results with these antibodies are similar to those with high performance liquid chromatography, a specific method in which cyclosporin is separated from its metabolites as part of the assay procedure. Because sample preparation and assay technique are more complicated with high performance liquid chromatography it is not as widely used as radioimmunoassay.

Cyclosporin

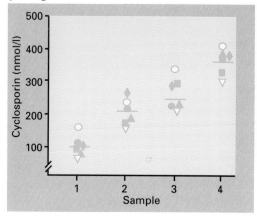

Results of measuring the whole blood cyclosporin concentrations in the same four samples in five different laboratories all using radioimmunoassay.

Criteria for measurement

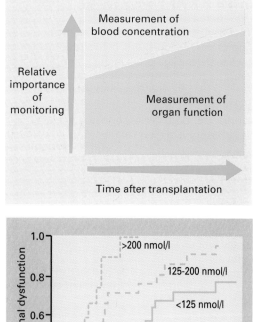

Risk of renal damage in patients receiving cyclosporin after bone marrow transplantation rises with higher cyclosporin concentrations (measured by radioimmunoassay of serum samples).

- The therapeutic range depends on the laboratory making the measurement and on the time after the start of treatment

- The risk of transplant rejection during the first six months of therapy increases at whole blood concentrations below 80-200 nmol/l (100-250 ng/ml)

- The risk of adverse effects increases at whole blood concentrations above 170-330 nmol/l (200-400 ng/ml)

Interpretation of results

The following discussion is based on measurements in whole blood. Those who use concentration measurements should know what type of assay and what type of sample matrix their local laboratory prefers and learn the target concentration ranges applicable to that laboratory, since these will differ among assays and types of sample. This in turn implies that each laboratory should, if possible, establish its own therapeutic and toxic concentration ranges based on patients in its catchment area.

We will now apply to cyclosporin the criteria which must be fulfilled in part or in full before the measurement of its plasma concentration in organ transplantation can be considered worth while.

Is there difficulty in interpreting clinical evidence of the therapeutic or toxic effects?

Information about the relation between blood concentrations of cyclosporin and its therapeutic effects is largely limited to its use in preventing the rejection of transplanted organs, although information about toxicity may relate to all of its clinical uses.

During the early stages after organ transplantation, when the risk of rejection is high, detecting evidence of rejection can be difficult, and since prediction of blood cyclosporin concentrations is limited by the enormous variability in the drug's kinetics, at this stage their measurement may be of use in determining an effective dose and in minimising the risk of toxicity. In the later stages, when the risk of rejection is lower and organ function tests better reflect the risk of rejection, measurements are needed less often.

In the special case of kidney transplantation, however, it may be impossible at every stage to use renal function tests to distinguish between an episode of transplant rejection on the one hand and cyclosporin induced renal damage on the other. In these cases measuring the blood cyclosporin concentration may be of value.

Is there a good relation between the blood concentration and its therapeutic or toxic effects?

In individual studies the therapeutic effects of cyclosporin correlate quite well with its effects in suppressing acute transplant rejection. However, when different studies are compared there is a wide variation in the cyclosporin concentration below which the risk of transplant rejection is increased. This variation in the relation between effect and concentration is largely due to differences between assay methods, although there may also be differences attributable to the time after transplantation.

If one of the more specific assay methods for cyclosporin is used (such as high performance liquid chromatography or a specific radioimmunoassay based on a monoclonal antibody) the risk of transplant rejection in the first six months seems to be increased when the trough whole blood cyclosporin concentration is below 80-200 nmol/l (100-250 ng/ml), depending on the laboratory. After six months lower concentrations may be compatible with maintained efficacy.

There is little information on the relation between the therapeutic response in psoriasis and the whole blood cyclosporin concentration, but there is some evidence that the two are not well related.

The risk of toxic effects increases with whole blood cyclosporin concentration, although there is a great deal of overlap with therapeutic concentrations. The risks of nephrotoxicity, hepatotoxicity, and other adverse effects increase at whole blood cyclosporin concentrations above 170-330 nmol/l (200-400 ng/ml), depending on the laboratory.

Is cyclosporin metabolised to active metabolites?

Cyclosporin is metabolised to several compounds, some of which may have therapeutic or toxic effects. However, their contribution to the actions of cyclosporin is probably less than 20 per cent. The use of specific assays allows these metabolites to be ignored but it is not currently known how important their activity is in treatment.

Factors affecting the blood concentration

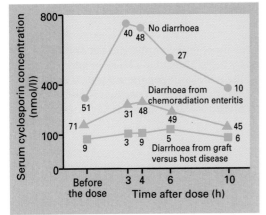

Cyclosporin absorption varies depending on the presence or absence of diarrhoea.

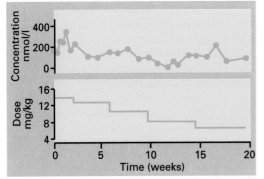

During long term therapy the dosage of cyclosporin can be reduced without affecting the plasma concentration.

The differences in distribution which can affect blood cyclosporin concentrations have been mentioned above. The following factors can also alter the blood concentration of cyclosporin for a given dose:

Altered absorption

Absorption of cyclosporin from the gastrointestinal tract is highly variable, but on average poor (about 30%). It is affected by gastrointestinal motility, and in particular by diarrhoea, which can cause reduced absorption.

Absorption also depends on the presence of bile salts. If the secretion of bile is reduced (for example, in severe liver disease or after liver transplantation) or if the bile is drained externally, the absorption of cyclosporin decreases. When there is external drainage of bile, clamping the T-tube may cause a fivefold rise in cyclosporin concentrations, and in patients with external drainage of bile, cyclosporin is often given intravenously.

After transplantation the systemic availability of cyclosporin seems to increase with duration of therapy, and after about three months lower dosages may result in the same steady state concentrations. This may be due to increased absorption from the gut or reduced first pass metabolism by the liver, or both.

Altered elimination

When liver function is severely impaired the clearance of cyclosporin is also reduced because of reduced enzyme activity and reduced blood flow through the liver.

The elimination of cyclosporin is faster in children than in adults.

Because cyclosporin is metabolised by enzymes of the cytochrome P450 group, its metabolism may be inhibited by enzyme inhibitors such as ketoconazole, cimetidine, and erythromycin and increased by enzyme inducers such as rifampicin, phenytoin, and carbamazepine.

Factors affecting interpretation

> Other nephrotoxic drugs may enhance the nephrotoxicity of cyclosporin

The blood concentration of cyclosporin at which nephrotoxicity may occur is altered by the presence of other nephrotoxic drugs, such as amphotericin and aminoglycoside antibiotics.

Use of blood concentrations

Case history: treatment of rejection soon after transplantation

A 48 year old man with chronic kidney failure had a kidney transplant. He had a good initial response and after loading doses of triple drug therapy was given oral maintenance dosages (azathioprine 1 mg/kg/day, prednisolone 1 mg/kg/day, and cyclosporin 8 mg/kg/day orally).

Ten days after transplantation he became acutely unwell with a Gram negative septicaemia, which was treated with ampicillin and gentamicin. His renal function deteriorated. His serum gentamicin concentrations were in the acceptable ranges (see chapter on aminoglycoside antibiotics), but his whole blood cyclosporin concentration was low at 65 nmol/l (80 ng/ml). A biopsy specimen of the transplanted kidney showed evidence of early rejection and he was treated with intravenous methylprednisolone (1 g intravenously for three days). He made a good recovery from his septicaemia. His dose of cyclosporin was then increased to 10 mg/kg/day and he subsequently remained well.

Conclusion

The measurement of the whole blood cyclosporin concentration did not change the immediate management of acute rejection (diagnosed by biopsy), but it did show that rejection was associated with undertreatment with cyclosporin and allowed a subsequent increase in dosage.

At the start of treatment with cyclosporin after organ transplantation, when the therapeutic dosage in a patient is not yet known, measurement of cyclosporin concentration is necessary in adjusting the dosage in order to achieve a target concentration. It is usual during this stage to measure the concentration every two days until a satisfactory concentration is achieved, and this usually takes about two weeks. Thereafter the concentration should be measured during an episode suggestive of rejection. In kidney transplantation this is particularly important in order to differentiate between rejection and inadequate treatment.

During longer term treatment monitoring is generally best carried out by measuring organ function (for example, creatinine clearance in a kidney transplant). However, if it is thought necessary to reduce the dosage of cyclosporin (after about three to six months), when lower target concentrations may be acceptable, dosages may be altered with the aid of blood concentration measurement.

Cyclosporin

Case history: cyclosporin toxicity

A 36 year old man who had had a successful hepatic transplantation had deteriorating renal function and a high whole blood cyclosporin concentration (250 nmol/l) (300 ng/ml). His renal function improved when the dosage of cyclosporin was reduced.

Conclusion

This case differs from the first case in that rejection was not a possible cause of the deterioration in renal function. The whole blood cyclosporin concentration suggested that cyclosporin toxicity was the cause, and kidney biopsy was not necessary.

If toxicity is suspected at any time, or if compliance is in doubt, blood cyclosporin measurements may help. They may also be helpful when an external bile drainage tube is clamped after hepatic surgery, if chronic diarrhoea develops (for example, during graft versus host disease after marrow transplantation), or when potentially interacting drugs are introduced or withdrawn.

Case history: deteriorating renal function during long term treatment after transplantation

A 29 year old woman who had had a successful kidney transplantation four months before, developed gradually deteriorating renal function. Cyclosporin was undetectable in a whole blood sample, and it transpired that she had been distressed by facial hypertrichosis and had stopped taking cyclosporin. When the risks of non-compliance were explained to her she restarted treatment and her renal function did not deteriorate further.

Conclusion

This case illustrates the usefulness of measuring blood drug concentrations in diagnosing poor compliance.

If the dosage of cyclosporin is changed at any time the blood concentration should be checked again two days later, by which time a steady state should have been reached. In patients in whom the half life is prolonged (for example, in liver disease) it takes longer to reach steady state.

As with the monitoring of any drug by measurement of plasma concentration, it is important to interpret the blood cyclosporin concentration in the light of the patient's clinical condition. For example, if there is evidence of good transplant function during long term treatment you would not necessarily adjust the dosage of cyclosporin simply to ensure that the blood concentration falls within some notional target range.

Timing of measurement

All of the above advice relates to trough concentration measurements (measurements made in samples taken just before the next dose is due).

Cyclosporin measurements should be made before the next dose, at the same time of day on each occasion

---

Because the pharmacokinetics of cyclosporin may be subject to some diurnal variation the blood sample should be taken at the same time of day in each patient. This is most simply done before the morning dose, whether the patient is taking cyclosporin once or twice daily.

The sources of the data presented in the graphs are: B M Frey *et al, Transplantation Proceedings* 1987;**19**:1713-4 for results from five different laboratories; G C Yee *et al, Transplantation Proceedings* 1986;**18**:774-6 for probability of renal dysfunction *v* days of treatment; Atkinson *et al, Br J Haematology* 1984;**56**:223-31 for absorption with and without diarrhoea; and F Sjöqvist, *Proceedings of the Second World Conference on Clinical Pharmacology and Therapeutics,* American Society for Pharmacology and Experimental Therapeutics, 1983:38 for plasma concentration with duration of treatment. The data are reproduced with permission of the journals.

MAKING THE MOST OF PLASMA DRUG CONCENTRATION MEASUREMENTS

D J M Reynolds, J K Aronson

> **Criteria that a drug should satisfy for plasma concentration measurements to be useful**
> - Difficulty in interpreting clinical evidence of therapeutic or toxic effects
> - A good relation between the plasma drug concentration and the therapeutic or toxic effect, or both
> - A low toxic:therapeutic ratio
> - Is not metabolised to important active metabolites

In the previous chapters we have outlined the principles of monitoring drug therapy by measuring the plasma drug concentration and shown how they can be applied to specific drugs (digoxin, lithium, theophylline, phenytoin, aminoglycoside antibiotics, and cyclosporin), for which the criteria in the box are sufficiently fulfilled to justify monitoring.

Usefulness of measurement

When the criteria are not rigorously met the regular use of plasma drug concentration measurements is hard to justify. None the less, measurements are sometimes made for other drugs, including anticonvulsants such as carbamazepine and ethosuximide; antiarrhythmic drugs; tricyclic antidepressants; anti-infective drugs such as itraconazole, vancomycin, and flucytosine; and methotrexate. These are drugs which fulfil some but not all of the criteria. In some circumstances, however, their measurement may be helpful (for example, in monitoring compliance or in patients with renal failure).

Even for drugs that fulfil the criteria there is some controversy about the usefulness of monitoring their plasma concentrations.

> **Indications for measuring plasma drug concentrations**
> - Monitoring compliance
> - Individualising therapy
>   —during early therapy
>   —during dosage changes
> - Diagnosing undertreatment
> - Avoiding toxicity
> - Diagnosing toxicity
> - Monitoring and detecting drug interactions
> - Guiding withdrawal of therapy

Firstly, it has been argued that there is no good evidence that targeting plasma concentrations improves the therapeutic outcome[1 2] and that the hypothesis that it is of therapeutic value needs to be tested.[3] These arguments ignore the axiom that implies that there is a better relation between concentration and effect than between dose and effect. Thus it should be possible to improve therapy with a drug by monitoring its plasma concentrations. In practice, however, the benefit to be gained is likely to be small when the drug does not fulfil the necessary criteria. There is certainly a need for prospective studies to determine the benefit of monitoring drug concentrations, though there would be considerable practical and ethical difficulties in designing such studies.

Secondly, it is argued that the value of the technique is reduced by problems in defining therapeutic ranges—for example, when there are conditions that alter a drug's pharmacodynamic effects.[2 3] But this argument merely emphasises the need for proper interpretation of plasma drug concentrations in these conditions.

> Treat the patient, not the plasma drug concentration

Thirdly, it has been said that too often it is the plasma concentration which is treated rather than the patient[4] and that much monitoring is rendered useless by, for example, inappropriate timing of sampling.[3] That this is so is evidence that plasma drug concentration monitoring is being misused rather than that it is of no use.

Making the most of plasma drug concentration measurements

There is no justification for routine measurements of plasma drug concentrations without a definite purpose. For example, in an epileptic patient taking phenytoin who is free of fits and is otherwise well routine measurement is of little value and indeed may lead to inappropriate adjustments of dosage. However, it may be of value when, for example, an interacting drug is introduced or when a dosage adjustment is required in a patient whose fits are poorly controlled.

The indirect benefits of measuring the plasma drug concentration include education of the doctor in the principles underlying dose responsiveness and the detection of important new drug interactions.[1] The use of such measurements in research is outside the scope of this book.

How to use the measurements properly

Timing of blood samples

Aminoglycoside antibiotics
  Intravenous: Peak—15 min after the end of an intravenous infusion; trough—just before the next dose
  Intramuscular or intravenous bolus: Peak—1 h after the injection; trough—just before the next dose
Cyclosporin—Just before the next dose; measure at the same time of day on each occasion (for example, before the morning dose)
Digoxin—At least 6 h after the last dose (it is therefore best to give a single daily dose in the evening)
Lithium—12 h after the last dose
Phenytoin—Timing is not important
Theophylline
  During an infusion: 4-6 h after starting the infusion; stop infusion for 15 min before taking the sample
  Oral: just before the next dose; measure at the same time of day on each occasion

Types of samples required

Drug	Type of sample
Digoxin, phenytoin, theophylline	Plasma or serum
Aminoglycoside antibiotics, lithium	Serum
Cyclosporin	Whole blood or plasma (consult your laboratory)

Examples of interpreting low plasma drug concentrations

1 *Patient with atrial fibrillation taking digoxin*
Ventricular rate=75 beats/min
Plasma digoxin concentration=0·6 nmol/l

Discussion—It would be better to withdraw the drug than to increase the dosage to achieve a "therapeutic" plasma concentration as it is unlikely that digoxin at such a low plasma concentration is contributing to slowing the heart rate. Withdrawal is unlikely to result in deterioration

2 *Patient taking phenytoin*
Patient with epilepsy, free of fits for 12 months. Plasma phenytoin concentration= 25 μmol/l

Discussion—There may be therapeutic benefit in patients with plasma concentrations below the therapeutic range and withdrawal may lead to recurrence of fits. Treatment should probably be continued.

If plasma drug concentration measurements are to be of any value attention must be paid to the timing of blood sampling, the type of blood sample, the measurement technique, and interpretation of the result.

Timing of sampling

It is important to take the blood sample for drug measurement at the correct time after dosing. This has been dealt with for each drug in previous chapters, and the appropriate timings are summarised in the box. Errors in timing are probably responsible for the greatest number of errors in interpreting results.

Types of samples

For most drugs the blood sample can be taken into a heparinised tube or allowed to clot, and there are no important restrictions on storage before measurement. For lithium and aminoglycosides, however, samples should be allowed to clot and separated within an hour. For cyclosporin it is important to consult the local laboratory for details on sampling technique.

Measurement technique

For the laboratory's part it is important to ensure that the assay used is as reliable and specific as possible and that appropriate quality control is undertaken. Assay results should be available quickly and preferably within 24 hours of receiving the sample, as the most important uses of measurement are during dosage adjustments and in diagnosing toxicity, when rapid decisions need to be made. Indeed, there is evidence that on site measurement of antiepileptic drugs has an immediate impact on clinical decision making.[5]

Interpretation of the result

The most important principle in interpreting the plasma drug concentration is that the treatment should be tailored to the patient's needs. In doing so you should take into account not only the concentration but also other clinical features that may affect the relation between concentration and effect. It would be wrong to use the concentration measurement in isolation and to try to engineer the plasma concentration into a predetermined range (see examples in the box). It is important therefore for the doctor responsible to know how to interpret the result in the light of the patient's condition.

Indications for measurement

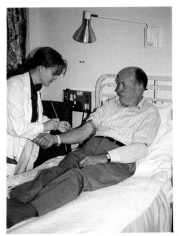

Measuring the plasma drug concentration may be useful in individualising treatment.

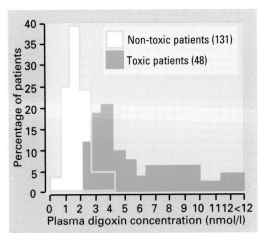

Measuring the plasma digoxin concentration may be helpful in confirming the diagnosis of toxicity.

Examples of factors that affect target ranges for plasma drug concentrations

Drug	Factor
Aminoglycoside antibiotics	Other nephrotoxic drugs (enhance the risk of renal damage)
Cyclosporin	Other nephrotoxic drugs (enhance the risk of renal damage)
Digoxin	Potassium depletion
Lithium	Electroconvulsive therapy (may enhance the action of lithium)
Phenytoin	Altered protein binding (for example, in chronic renal failure)

Making the most of plasma drug concentration measurements

There are several circumstances in which plasma drug concentration measurement may be helpful, although each indication does not apply equally to each drug.

Compliance—In the chapter on compliance we discussed the ways in which compliance may be monitored. Measuring the plasma concentration may be helpful as a low measurement reflects either poor recent compliance or undertreatment. Poor compliance is implicated if the patient is taking a dose which is unlikely to be associated with such a low concentration or if previous measurements suggest that the plasma concentration should be higher for the given dose.

Individualising therapy—When starting drug therapy it may be useful to measure the plasma concentration in order to tailor the dosage to the individual. This applies to all drugs, although it is most important for lithium, cyclosporin, and the aminoglycoside antibiotics. If for any reason at a later stage the dosage regimen has to be altered (for example, in patients with renal failure) plasma concentration measurement may again be helpful.

Diagnosing undertreatment—Undertreatment of an established condition may often be diagnosed on observing a poor clinical response. However, when the drug is being used as prophylaxis you cannot observe the response and may have to settle for giving a dosage that will produce a target plasma concentration. This applies particularly to lithium in preventing manic depressive attacks, to phenytoin in preventing fits and to cyclosporin in preventing transplant rejection.

Avoiding toxicity—In all cases measurement during the early stages of treatment allows you to avoid plasma concentrations likely to be associated with toxicity.

Diagnosing toxicity—In many cases drug toxicity can be diagnosed clinically. For example, it is usually easy to recognise acute phenytoin toxicity, and measuring the plasma concentration may not be necessary for the diagnosis, although it may be helpful in adjusting the dosage subsequently. On the other hand, digoxin toxicity may mimic some of the effects of heart disease, and measuring the plasma concentration in cases in which toxicity is suspected may be helpful in confirming the diagnosis. Similarly, nephrotoxicity due to aminoglycoside antibiotics is hard to distinguish clinically from that caused by a severe generalised infection, and the plasma concentration may help to distinguish the two.

Drug interactions—If a potentially interacting drug is added measurement of the plasma concentration may guide subsequent changes in dosage. For example, when giving a thiazide diuretic to a patient taking lithium, measurement of the plasma lithium concentration will help to avoid toxicity. This also applies to theophylline when erythromycin is added. Conversely, measurement of the whole blood cyclosporin concentration will help to avoid undertreatment if rifampicin is added.

Stopping treatment—Measurement of the plasma drug concentration may guide when to stop treatment in two circumstances.

(1) When the plasma concentration is below the therapeutic range in a well patient. For example, if the plasma digoxin concentration is below the therapeutic range in a patient whose clinical condition is satisfactory then withdrawal of digoxin is unlikely to lead to clinical deterioration. Note that this use of the plasma concentration measurement depends on the concept that there is a lower end to the therapeutic range. This is not always the case—while it is probably true for digoxin it is not true for other drugs, particularly phenytoin (see box on previous page).

(2) When the plasma concentration is high without therapeutic benefit. For example, if there is no response to lithium and the serum concentration is at the upper end of the therapeutic range increased dosage is unlikely to be beneficial and the risk of toxicity is high. Withdrawal of lithium and the use of different treatment would be justified.

Making the most of plasma drug concentration measurements
Conclusions

Therapeutic and toxic plasma concentrations of commonly measured drugs

Drug	Concentration below which a therapeutic effect is unlikely	Concentration above which a toxic effect is more likely
Aminoglycosides:		
Amikacin	34 µmol/l (20 µg/ml) (at peak)	55 µmol/l (32 µg/ml) (at peak) 17 µmol/l (10 µg/ml) (at trough)
Gentamicin	5 µg/ml (at peak)†	12 µg/ml (at peak) 2 µg/ml (at trough)
Kanamycin	50 µmol/l (25 µg/ml) (at peak)	80 µmol/l (40 µg/ml) (at peak) 20 µmol/l (10 µg/ml) (at trough)
Cardiac glycosides:		
Digitoxin	20 nmol/l (15 ng/ml)	39 nmol/l (30 ng/ml)
Digoxin	1·0 nmol/l (0·8 ng/ml)	3·8 nmol/l (3 ng/ml)
Cyclosporin*	80-200 nmol/l (100-250 ng/ml)	170-330 nmol/l (200-400 ng/ml)
Lithium	0·4 mmol/l	1·0 mmol/l
Phenytoin	40 µmol/l (10 µg/ml)	80 µmol/l (20 µg/ml)
Theophylline	55 µmol/l (10 µg/ml)	110 µmol/l (20 µg/ml)

*Measured in whole blood by specific radioimmunoassay or high performance liquid chromatography. The actual results depend on the laboratory in which the measurement is made.

†This value may be lower if a synergistic antibiotic, such as penicillin, is being used concurrently.

In this book we have outlined the uses of measuring the plasma concentrations of some drugs and given guidelines on how such measurements should be made and interpreted.

The box summarises the target plasma concentrations for each of the drugs. In each case there is a concentration below which a therapeutic effect is unlikely and a concentration above which the risk of toxicity is high. These two concentrations imply a therapeutic range for each drug, but remember that there are circumstances in which strict adherence to a range of this kind is inappropriate. The plasma concentration should always be interpreted in the light of factors which may alter the effective therapeutic range.

Nor is it always necessary to measure plasma concentrations to achieve satisfactory drug therapy. Routine measurement without a clear purpose is as bad as no measurement at all. The application of the principles we have outlined should allow the rational use of plasma concentration measurement in optimising drug therapy.

1 Vozeh S. Cost-effectiveness of therapeutic drug monitoring. *Clin Pharmacokin* 1987;**13**:131-40.
2 Spector R, Park GD, Johnson GF, Vesell ES. Therapeutic drug monitoring. *Clin Pharmacol Ther* 1988;**43**:345-53.
3 McInnes GT. The value of therapeutic drug monitoring to the practising physician—an hypothesis in need of testing. *Br J Clin Pharmacol* 1989;**27**:281-4.
4 Sjöqvist F. Interindividual differences in drug responses: an overview. In: Rowland M, Sheiner LB, Steimer JL, eds. *Variability in drug therapy*. New York: Raven Press, 1985:1-10.
5 Larkin JG, Herrick AL, McGuire GM, Percy-Robb IW, Brodie MJ. Antiepileptic drug monitoring at the epilepsy clinic: a prospective evaluation. *Epilepsia* 1991;**32**:89-95.

INDEX

Index